Mental He~~a~~

2: About Diagnosis & Treatment

a jargon-free self training guide

MARIANNE RICHARDS

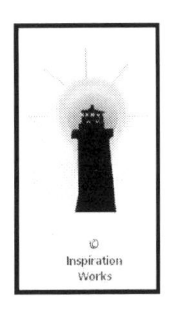

Copyright © 2017 Marianne Richards
All rights reserved.
www.InspirationWorks4U.co.uk

Mental Health Awareness
2: About Diagnosis & Treatment

© Marianne Richards 2017

ISBN-10: 154546782X
ISBN-13: 978-1545467824

InspirationWorks4U.co.uk

Printed in the USA by CreateSpace for InspirationWorks4U.co.uk
Cover design by Mole Graphics

All rights reserved. No part of this publication may be reproduced in a retrieval system or transmitted by any means, electronic or mechanical, photocopying or otherwise, without the prior permission of the copyright holders.

Whilst every effort has been made to ensure that the information contained within this book is correct at the time of going to press, the author and publisher can take no responsibility for the errors or omissions contained within.

DEDICATION

Tim. RIP

CONTENTS

		Pge
	Introduction	9
	The Bridge	11
	Acknowledgements	12

WHAT IS MENTAL ILLNESS

1	Who are the mentally ill?	13
2	Mental Illness & Community - Overview	19
3	Learning About Mental Illness - My Journey	27

DIAGNOSIS

4	Pre-Diagnosis – Moral and Social Issues	35
5	Diagnosing Mental Illness – Medical Model	43
6	Major Mental Illnesses - symptoms	47

TREATMENT OF MENTAL ILLNESS

7	Medical & Nursing Professionals	67
8	Non Medical Professionals	73
9	Talking Cures	81
10	Year 2000: Disagreement over Training Changes	93
11	Aftercare	103
12	Evidence v Experience	109
13	Graduate Mental Health Workers	115
14	Alternative & Complementary for Stress	119

CASE STUDIES

| 15 | Range of Case Studies | 123 |

	Appendix 1: Dr Parenti's Paper	131
	Glossary	139
	Further Reading	149
	Index	155

DIAGRAMS

Figure		Pge
	Headlines	13
1	Moral Panics	15
2	Mental Health /Illness Continuum	16
3	Cradle Song	21
4	Triggers of Mental Illness – Community Life	25
5	Continuum – Mental Health to Mental Illness	29
6	Parallel Experience	31
7	Woman with Mania – Bethlem Hospital	51
8	Phobia	55
9	Answers To Diagnostic Exercise	60
10	Overview: Types of Treatment	63
11	Cognitive Triangle	83
12	Change; Prochaska/ DiClemente model	95
13	Group Behaviour in Change Situations	97
14	Lewin's Unified Field Theory	99
15	We Must Never Forget Asylum Patients	105
16	Therapeutic Communities	107
17	SCIE Services	113
18	Sources of Self Help and After Care	117
19	Social Problems of Mental Illness	159

'Words don't just reflect reality, they create reality.'
Jose Silva, Silva Mind Control

INTRODUCTION

Volume 1 of this series contains a brief history of mental illness, a backcloth of the legislation and how patients /the community view each other (stigmatization). You cannot understand mental illness without knowing its social and historic context, so I urge you to read volume one.

This volume covers diagnosis, treatment and the professionals involved in mental healthcare. There are a selection of case histories and some diagnostic exercises. Do remember, never go outside your professional competence. These exercises are to give you an idea how mental health diagnoses are made, and are not intended to form all or part of any formal training.

Many patients are now eschewing medicine in favour of treatments which stem from ancient Eastern traditions. In a world rocked by change it seems we are seeking stress relief and understanding, rather than medication. It is interesting that mindfulness and brief therapy are now accepted treatments for mild to moderate depression.

A note of caution; there is often no researched evidence, so always suggest to patients they exercise precaution, as there are many charlatans about. However, some treatments have anecdotal evidence as being effective for stress.

Welcome to my book and I hope you enjoy reading about the fascinating field you have chosen to study.

Marianne C Richards
October 2017

The Bridge

Sitting by your side
I try to find the words.
They will not come.

I catch your eye
You catch mine.
I hold out my hand.
You take it.

A bridge is forged.

I hold your hand
As the sky is falling
The sky is falling.

I will hold your hand
Though the sky is falling
The sky is falling.

    MCR
    Aug 1992

ACKNOWLEDGEMENTS

I would like to thank the following
- ♥ National Institute for Health & Clinical Excellence
- ♥ The British Film Institute
- ♥ my reviewers
- ♥ University of Bath

Copyright Permissions

Text
Crown copyright material is reproduced with the permission of the Controller of HMSO and the Queen's Printer for Scotland.

Images

Photographs The following images [figure no + image reference] supplied by Wellcome Picture Library, under Creative Commons License http://wellcomeimages.org/. None of these images has been altered. Woman with Mania fig V0029627, Asylum patients original title 'types of insanity' fig L0006935.

Illustrations by Mole Graphics.

Photographs of St John's Hospital by the author. These are held in joint copyright with the Buckinghamshire Collection, Aylesbury.

NOTES:
The opinions expressed in this book belong to the author and do not reflect the views of any organisation, agency, publisher or the reviewers.

If we have inadvertently breached any copyrights, please contact us via the website and we herewith apologise and promise to put it right in future editions.

'In the country of the blind, the one-eyed man is king.'
Erasmus (1466-1536); also H G Wells. The Country of the Blind.

1 WHO ARE THE MENTALLY ILL?

Content
Country of the Blind
Criminality & Mental Illness
Who Are the Mentally Ill
Does Insanity Exist?
How Do we define insanity
Personal experience of Psychosis

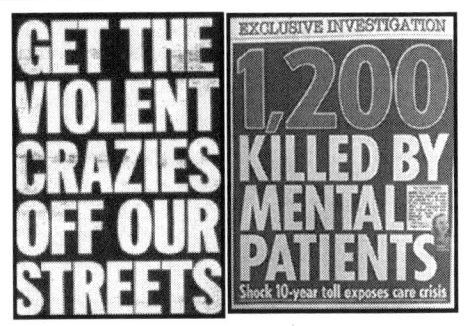

http://www.theguardian.com/society/reality-check/2013/oct/07/sun-people-killed-mental-health-true

Country of the Blind

It seems we still live in the country of the blind. In the 20th century but less so now, there were a spate of moral panics fuelled by lurid headlines (figure 1). In the public eye, criminal acts committed by people with paranoid schizophrenia or psychopathic personality disorder, are taken to be indicative of everyone with enduring mental illness. In fact, murders committed by the forensically insane are far less in number than those committed by criminals who are wicked by choice. Bad press precludes empathy for mental illness in general. Although their behaviour defied moral codes, none of these men were ruled to be criminally insane:

- Eric Harris and Dylan Klebold - assassinated 13 innocent young students at Columbine High School, America
- Harold Shipman – GP who poisoned an unknown number of his patients. Over 887 deaths were investigated in the public enquiry of which he is suspected of killing at least 260.
- Armin Meiwes – cannibal, who advertised for a willing victim on the internet and found one in Bernd Jurgen Brandes. Meiwes was eventually imprisoned for murder but not considered insane.

There is a key difference between breaking moral codes and/or the law in a state of sanity or doing the same during an episode of mental illness. The difference is intent. Whilst the above people deliberately set out to murder for their own reasons, they were found to be sane when they made this decision. In the case of psychopathic killer Ian Brady, he was guilty on the one hand [moral justice] but being born without that part of the brain that allows reason, he was sent to a hospital to the criminally insane.

Criminality & Mental Illness
Links between criminality and mental illness are the subject of continuing debate as are the boundaries between what is considered normal behaviour and morality in 21st century life.

Who Are the Mentally Ill
All mental health workers should be aware that all of us suffer stress and nearly 25% of the population will be diagnosed with a mental illness at some point. I find it amusing that of many mental health workers I am one of few who can prove I am sane – because I have been discharged from a mental hospital. So-called normal members of the public have generally not had this test applied.

Illness of the mind is a common experience, not something that afflicts some imagined sub species of human beings. The only reason you will not know this is that too many people, including professionals, are frightened of admitting symptoms. In the NHS particularly, it is clearly frowned upon for mental health professionals to admit to being occasionally insane or sometimes afflicted with minor mental illness, as if somehow that denigrates their position. This hypocrisy adds to stigma, in my view and also degrades the status of patients such people work with.

1:4 people will be diagnosed with depressive illness and 1:25 with schizophrenia. Many more will attend GP's for physical symptoms that are known to be connected with mental distress: skin problems, backache, physical aches and tiredness.

So why is it that people seemingly happy to talk to a GP about intimate body parts but reluctant to talk about emotional problems, disturbances to perception (e.g. hallucinations - more common than you might think) or any other signs of 'going mad'. You might discuss these with a close friend but talking outside the family is taboo. In the USA, people do not appear to have this problem and a visit to a psychiatrist is more likely to trigger a request for his / her contact details than a negative reaction.

I believe there are many answers, including fear, lack of education about mental illnesses, stigmatization, bad press, fear of prognosis, shame. There is also a strong perceived link between mental illness and attacks on the public, such as the sort of headlines you used to read in the tabloids "Crazy axe murderer killer gets life" or "young actress in suicide bid" or "schizo gets life". Ignorance about the meaning of mental illness, the facts of its control or cure maintains stigmatization.

figure 1 Moral Panics

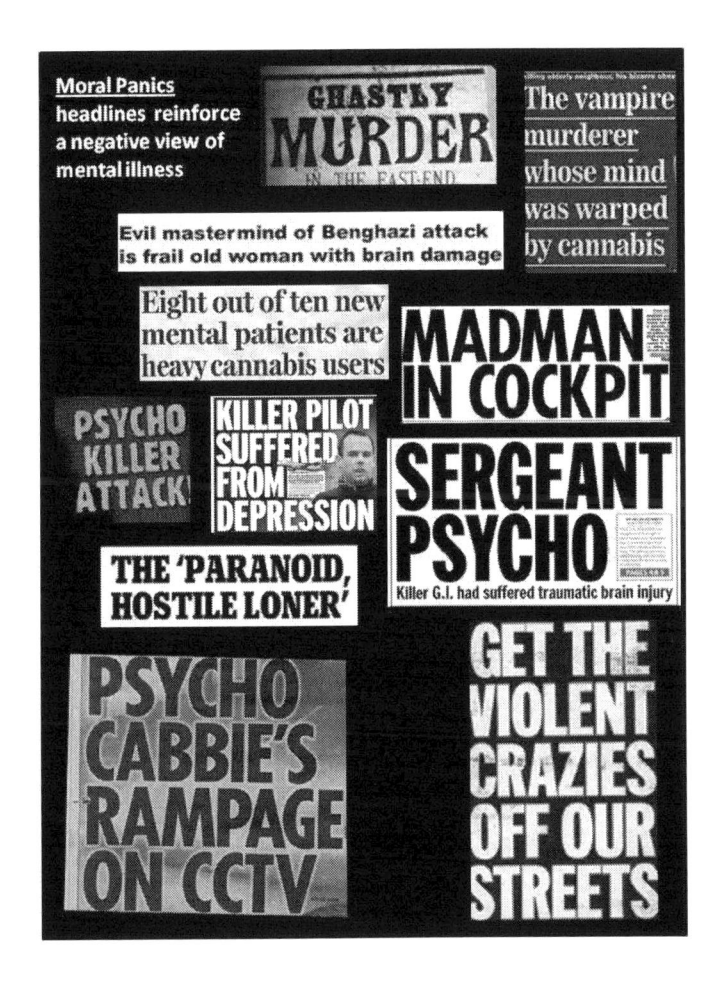

Even in the 21st century with our information overload, a most of the public learn about mental illness only through sensational headlines. Thankfully this is changing, thanks to liaison between the media and the Royal College of Psychiatrists and education in schools. Far more murders are committed by so-called sane than mentally ill persons. There are very few forms of mental illness which lead to murderous/socially repugnant behaviour; among them, psychopathic personality disorder, paranoid schizophrenia, paraphilia or paedophilia. And even among patients with these diagnoses, a still lesser number go on to commit crimes. The borderline between forensic mental illness and criminal activity is shifting with new medication, treatments and shifting moral values. The mad or bad debate continues and it is important to be aware of it.

Many professionals would not class stress as mental illness, but patients suffer stress as a result of their symptoms and the environment. Not only patients, but loved ones and carers too. If stress was classed as mental illness, the field might become less stigmatized, demonstrating a continuum from mental health to mental illness. Mental illness is more common than you might think: 1:4 people will become mentally ill during their life.

Figure 2   Mental Health / Mental Illness Continuum

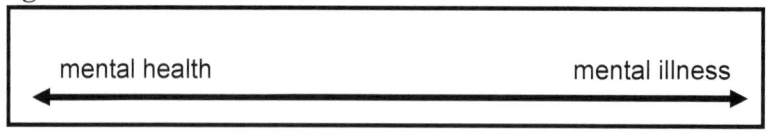

```
| mental health                          mental illness |
|  <------------------------------------------------->  |
```

Does Insanity exist?

Some professionals, even Psychiatrists, question whether sanity and insanity exist as states or whether they are social constructs. It is vital that mental health workers are not afraid to ask questions, even if they are challenging:
- do sanity and insanity exist
- how do we define mental illness
- how does mental illness present
- is mental illness a social or community construct

First, some questions about perception. The philosopher George Berkeley (1685-1753) asked, if no one hears a tree falling in the forest, does the sound of falling exist. I am going to pose you a question; does insanity exist, if there is no one to observe it?

Imagine a man alone on an island, a man who has views very different to your own and lives in a completely alien way. Could his extraordinary perceptions be considered sane. If someone with opposing perceptions joins him on the island, who is sane and who deluded - or are their realities both valid i.e. sane? In which case, how many people have to live on the island, before realities are accepted that then define sanity? One answer is, that no one can be certain, because no one possesses the power of entering someone else's mind to 'see' how they think. Or we could dismiss them as 'the island of the insane'. But what if they consider themselves sane, and your island mad?

Prisoners in solitary confinement often experience hallucinations. And friends of people thus isolated report that their friend now has different perceptions. Consider Pattie Hurst, millionaire Randolph Hurst's daughter, who was kidnapped by the Symbionese Liberation Army and months later willingly joined them to rob a bank and take part in extortion (see reading list). The phenomenon by which captives grow close to their kidnappers is call Stockholm Syndrome.

If you suggested to someone steeped in religious or mystical practice that their vision was a hallucination and should be treated with Haloperidol, that they had a mental health problem, then you would most certainly offend and horrify them.

How Do We Define Insanity

We could define 'going mad' as having extraordinary perceptions which other people do not share. But if this is true then the religious ecstasies reported by hermits or anchorites must surely be considered madness, rather than divine inspiration? The problem is one of perception. This is a profound question; you are not merely diagnosing but judging existential questions;

- whose reality is more real
- whose perception or spiritual nuances are valid
- and who decides?

Though it is difficult to define insanity, it is easier in practice to recognize. If someone is psychotic i.e. experience visual or auditory hallucinations (visions or sounds/voices that no one else shares), they are unlikely to live in what we call the real world safely. For their own protection, they must be hospitalized for treatment and carefully monitored, for their sake as well as the public.

Personal Experience of Psychosis

I have undergone two episodes of psychosis, the first the more horrific because it went undiagnosed. The first was during a traumatic divorce, the second a toxic psychosis after a breast operation. I continued somehow to work, but my then colleagues said I looked and acted differently. I recall the detail even now, decades on, and their fear and disgust at my physical state. My employer was a bully and prior to this was already trying to get rid of me, leaving notes on my desk every day about my 'attention to detail' slipping. his behaviour was also, I believe causal, and I was not the first female to receive his cavalier attitudes. (This was a forces housing association, where you would have thought there would be more empathy).

When I went to my GP and told him there was a man outside taking notes of everything we said, you would have thought he would have had me sectioned– but he merely looked very puzzled, so eventually I went home. I suppose he had no training and little experience of mental illness. Later I was informed I nearly did not survive the trauma, for this went on months, over a year, as day became night, there were moments of clarity followed by night visions and voices which occasionally return. All those years ago I went on suffering, but had I been given a choice, I would have taken medication. The point is, drawing the line is perhaps more difficult to describe than in practice, but knowing how difficult it is, is important.

Key Learning
- bad press – leads to moral panic, with the public viewing mental illness with fear and suspicion, i.e. they equate murderous states with mental illness, rather than understanding that most murders are committed by 'sane' persons who kill/maim with intent
- who are the mentally ill – any of us. mental illness is very common in the population
- fears – fears and stigma surround mental illness, leading to reluctance to seek diagnosis for mental symptoms (fear of stigma, perceived weakness, linking to bad press (as above)
- does insanity exist – consider the island, religious ecstasies
- what is insanity – open to question, except in the case of psychosis, where the patient is unlikely to survive for long without treatment
- it is easier to recognise insanity than describe it in another person but the point as mental health workers is to study the subject carefully

> 'To think otherwise than our contemporaries think is ... disturbing; it is even indecent, morbid or blasphemous, and therefore socially dangerous for the individual.'
> C G Jung, Modern Man in Search of a Soul

2   MENTAL ILLNESS & THE COMMUNITY - OVERVIEW

Content
Commonality of Mental Illness
Supposed Causes of Mental Illness:
    environment, genetics, cultural, life, attitudes
Perceptions About Mental Illness

To sum up the last chapter. On a desert island inhabited by two or three people it would be impossible to have a line between sanity and madness. There have to be a group, in order to measure what passes for sanity. If you volume 1, you might recall the ship of fools, an early practice of sending insane people to sea in the hope of being cured. Some such patients were in fact cured, although others died in misery far from home. On such a ship, are the patients or sailors insane? There are more patients than sailors..

Commonality of Mental Illness
The prevalence of mental illness is surprisingly high, with nearly 25% of the population liable to diagnosis at some point in their lives, about the same number who suffer the scourge of depressive illness. Given this prevalence, stigmatisation is absurd.

The overwhelming reason for stigmatisation is fear, due to lack of education about mental health. The Government stipulate that mental health education is taught in schools but a quick glance at the national curriculum shows this is not viewed as seriously as it might. There are no standards, in citizenship or health, advising what should be taught. When I checked with the Department for Health and Education, I was told this was left to individual schools. This is a glaring omission.

I went further, in explaining that everyone experiences some phenomena which could be taken for symptoms of mental illness. I gave the examples of bereavement and falling in love both of which trigger extreme emotional reaction; that it was common for people to have hallucinations of dead people [if recently bereaved]. This is why clinicians, particularly new ones, have to exercise extreme caution when using clinical terminology which labels people.

Supposed Causes of Mental Illness

No one knows the real cause of mental illness and probably we will never know because the issues are very complex. However, it is generally accepted these factors are involved:
- environment – birth, living conditions
- genetics, parental behaviour
- psychological make-up
- cultural issues, personal beliefs
- life events
- community attitude - acceptance factor

So there are internal and external factors. Some are set in stone (genetic factors) whilst others alter (attitude and environment). These factors do not work in isolation, but are linked e.g.
- life events affect individual psychology
- environment has an effect on cultural issues

Environment We have no control about the conditions under which we are born; area, class, parentage, relations, upbringing. However, as we grow up we begin to exercise choice as we separate from parental influences. Some people have traumatic early lives that may take decades to work through, if they recover at all. Others will transcend trauma to live rich, full lives. Some might live wonderful lives but when tragedy strikes, it strikes them the harder, being unprepared.

Genetics Although the genetic code has been broken by Francis, Wilkins, Watson and Crick, there is a long way to go before there is deep understanding of the links between genes and psychological makeup. We know the names of the proteins that form the building blocks of life and how they fit together, but cannot predict what a person will become – how their life will turn out. This is the meaning of my poem Cradle Song.

Psychological make-up – this is a complex issue. There is not only the genetic [birth] factor but the complexities of how a person learns to communicate with the world because of:
- their experiences [life events – what happens to them]
- their perceptions [how they view their experiences].

This is sometimes referred to as the nature versus nurture argument; whether upbringing or genetics is responsible for the resulting psychological profile of a person. Where I find this most interestingly played out is in the psychological profiles of serial killers and bullies.

figure 3

CRADLE SONG

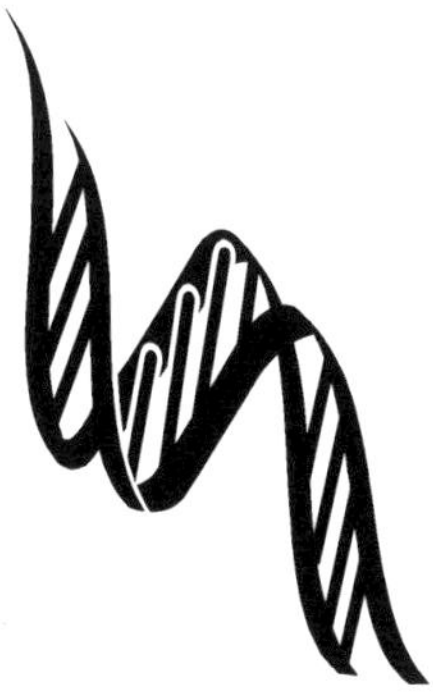

They say the secret's out, nothing left to know.
Franklin, Watson and Crick have written
The Book of Life, the definitive version -
DNA (the film of the book is on its way).

2.9 billion letters and 100,000 proteins
In synthesis - that's life in a nutshell.
Even then, the scientists say,
It can be boiled down a little bit more
We are made of just four proteins;
Adenine, Thymine, Cytosine, Guanine.

Silent, the baby sleeps in his cradle-
Warm, cream-parchment skin.
Tiny blank pages in an unwritten book.

Pale moonbeams slither on icy pavements
The frost shimmers like fragmented stars
The night-sky shivers in wispy robes of cloud.
As the womb-waters rocked, now the cradle rocks.

Child of my dreams, beloved son, cherished grandson.
Where will life take you? What will you become?
Adenine - the pioneer? Thymine - the scientist?
Cytosine - the artist? Guanine - the man of peace?
Womb to cradle. Cradle to ship. Ship's Captain.

All I can wish for you a fair wind with full sails
And fine weather. A sound and loyal crew.
Your mother's love and care. Strong arms to hold you.
A wise heart to guide you. A port in the storm.

Adenine the pioneer; Thymine the scientist
Cytosine the artist, Guanine the man of peace.

MCR Feb. 2004

Cultural issues – We have all witnessed how culture affects individuals and large groups for better or worse. This is exacerbated when an individual or group from one culture goes to live in a different environment and different culture. Of course, rivalry can be healthily played out on sports fields or in competitions, or discussed amicably. But stress comes on heavily when there are clashes between organised religions, gang cultures, or individuals of different natures in an unwelcoming community. Supporting an individual view often comes at risk in such places, to the individual and their family. Consider Moslem schoolgirl, Malala Yousafzai, shot in the head by the Taliban merely for going to school (she went on to win the Nobel prize for peace after defying them). It is a constant battle between those who desire something and those who thwart them; those open to change and zealots. All these are stress factors – the factor of fitting in, the factor of not wanting to stand out, wanting to carve an identity against the danger of raising your head above the parapet and being shot at (literally or figuratively).

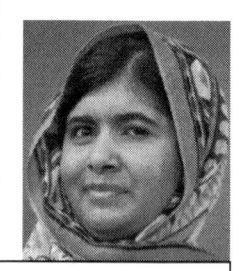

"I didn't want my future to be imprisoned in my four walls & just cooking & giving birth."

Stress caused by any of these community based difficulties can trigger symptoms of mental illness. Whether there are pre-existing genetic factors to receive this extra trigger, or whether the resulting mental illness comes from the environment alone, the result is the same. Later I will write of the difficulties of diagnosing someone from a different culture.

Life We cannot get away from life for better or worse. Experience and attitude shape our future. Our attitudes are linked with culture, genes and psychological makeup. Serial killers and saints originate from the same tree. More of that in another book. Life events are huge triggers for mental illness, whether through 'natural' trauma like bereavement or even birth, to psychosis caused by prolonged exposure to extreme stressors.

Community attitudes – I experienced at first hand a small community turning on someone. I have also been a target. Like tyrant children, communities can easily turn destructive if ill informed or lacking insight / control. But I have also seen individuals rise above circumstances. Living with supportive people makes a difference to those with mental health problems. But, sadly, attitudes often become triggers to symptoms in themselves. Look at the diagram, burdens of mental illness. The social factors are often overlooked or under estimated.

Perceptions of Individuals

Because I do not seek the company of others (as an autist, avoid it when I cant) I am often considered strange. But that does not mean I am mentally ill. yet these two are often equated. The attitude of the community towards those dingy closed curtains and a shadowy figure inside that never greet a neighbour is often a cause of worry or fear, but why?

Loners have been feared since early times and those who choose to live outside the confined box of expectations are less welcome than those who conform. Yet why are such people more likely to be considered mentally ill than the bank official with an expensive car and house, who is actually mediated for schizophrenia? One answer is perception. The other is lack of information or training. Here are a few examples:

- My brother mutters and is frequently scruffy but does not mean he needs medication because people are embarrassed. He is in fact highly intelligent but eccentric. He might have been burned or locked away in past times. And, for the record, I talk to myself in the street too.
- A charity worker was detained by a Sainsbury security guard, because he thought the young man was shoplifting. It turns out it was a scruffy charity worker doing his legitimate shopping.
- Anthony Worrall Thompson, the celebrity chef, admitted shoplifting, saying he needed help.
- Dr Harold Shipman became the most prolific serial killer of all time. He was diagnosed with a personality disorder. Shipman committed suicide.
- A scientist believes eternal life is not only possible but has a plan to advance this reality. Dr Aubrey de Grey, an intelligent computer expert, has been offered a large grant to research his beliefs.

Mental illness presents in many forms:
- conditions considered incurable
- conditions considered difficult to treat
- conditions relieved by medication or psychological treatment
- episodic conditions which affect behaviour, thinking or mood, which can be treated successfully and may or may not re-occur
- one off or occasional symptoms, triggered by life events

If patients present with organic disorders (cerebral palsy or Alzheimer's, head injury, Parkinsonism) with symptoms such as shaking, slurred speech, out-of-mind states, memory loss or hallucinations, modern practitioners attribute these to brain damage. We would not consider them curses of an angry god. In communities where mental illness is supposedly caused by angry gods, we might not be kind to the ill person, in case the gods wreak revenge on us. The modern equivalent seems to be jeering, stigmatizing or bullying. That which is not known is often feared.

Symptoms or Explainable Phenomena?

If we find it difficult to make assumptions about madness in the context of community then how much more difficult will it be in attempting to diagnose individuals when they come from another culture or community? We all have mental symptoms displayed as emotion or behaviour or perception so normality is very fleeting. If I enter a room and rush out without apparent reason could I be described a psychotic by an observer. This in fact happened, when I was being bullied by a colleague and observed by a Psychologist who, shall we say, forgot herself. If the observer had been informed I had mental illness, or was being bullied, these would have changed her perception. Misperceptions, especially by professionals, can be dangerous and profoundly damaging.

Stress Symptoms

Everyone has a mental symptoms, the most common being stress. Stress is not new but an ancient survival mechanism. I covered this in Understanding Mental Illness, the 2015 edition. Stress is a mental health symptom but not considered a major mental illness – though it can exacerbate existing conditions and trigger new ones, as I have written.

Basically, stress evolved as a way of readying us for fight/flight/freeze, according to the situation. Stress sends hormones rushing to the muscles, dumps waste matter (faeces and urine) to lighten our body, focuses the eyes, reduces focus on everything except the animal to be faced or run away from. But in modern times, we have no need for such activity, so the stress hormones build up, causing physical and mental symptoms. Remember, we are programmed:

- for survival, not to sit and fume in traffic or supermarket queues
- to kill or be killed, not act within social laws
- not to hold back feelings

Can you imagine the stress on a lion chained to a post starving, with a gazelle grazing 10 metres in front of him? Like apes in laboratory cages we have to comply with laws to survive and complicity costs us dear in the form of chained-up drives. An ape biting a scientist is a different matter to the experimenter torturing a lab animal. Every animal is affected by events:
1. a hungry lion chained becomes savage and dangerous
2. a man running down a road shouting about bees might be in pain from stings or under a delusion
3. a woman threatening an invisible presence might be experiencing hallucinations or being jilted via mobile phone

Figure 4 Burdens of mental illness

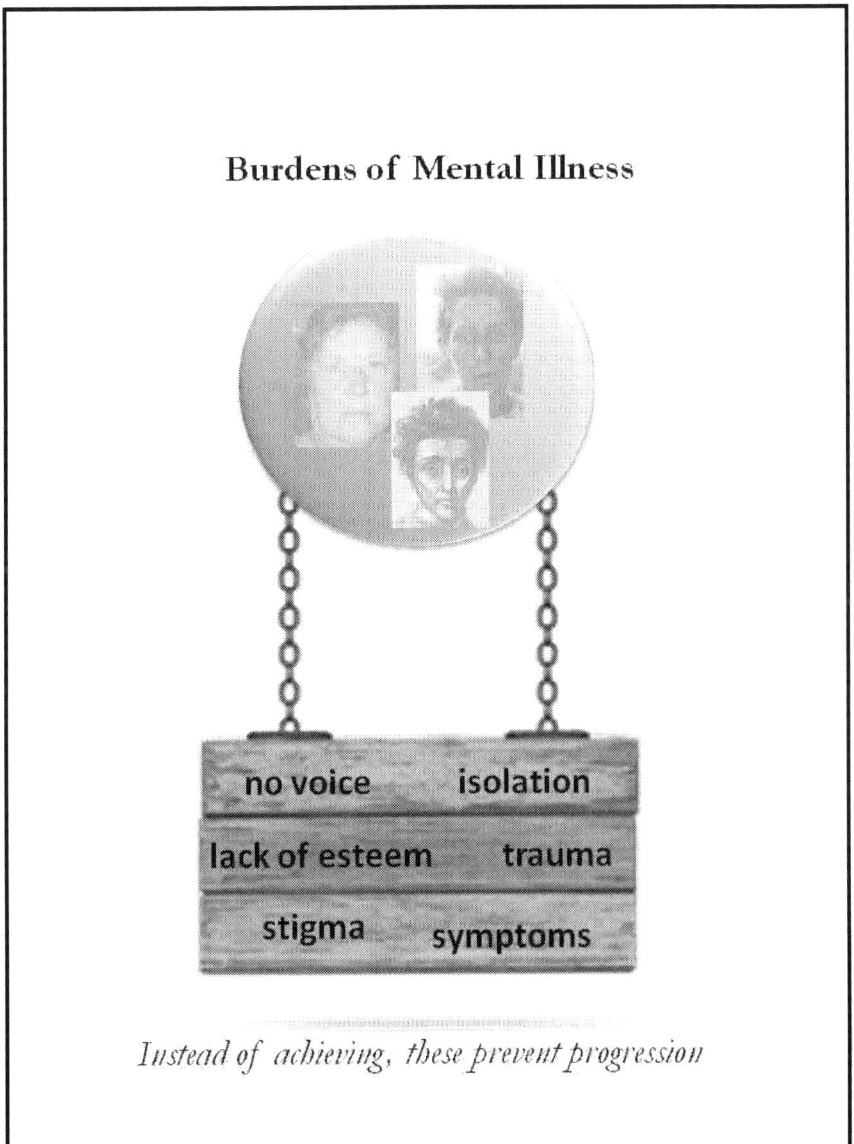

These situations resemble symptoms. However, given time, many symptoms resolve:
1. your lion, released from the stake, has his dinner and is sated
2. your stung man enjoys a pint whilst re-telling his tale.
3. the woman handbags her ex-boyfriend

So, stress IS a mental health worker's remit, even if it is not a mental illness. Stress can kill, stress exacerbates symptoms of mental illness and might trigger an episode. Stress affects most mental patients AND loved ones, carers. That is why many Trusts offer stress relief training courses.

Key Learning
- Diagnosis and Community **-** Diagnosis has little meaning outside a community setting. Consider the Island and the Ship of Fools.
- Commonality of Mental Illness - current figures show a quarter of the population is likely to become mentally ill during their lives.
- Misinterpreting Symptoms - it is easy to misperceive symptoms, when cultural, society and beliefs are not taken into consideration.
- Perceptions – eccentricity does not equate to mental illness, except in the eyes of the public
- Stress – is a huge factor in mental health patients, carers and loved ones. It can worsen / trigger existing conditions AND trigger new episodes of mental illness

How can one see the beauty of the day, when the mind and the heart and the brain are so clouded by the past as authority.'
Krishnamurti

3   LEARNING ABOUT MENTAL ILLNESS - MY JOURNEY

Content
On Learning
Why Do We Become Analytical?
Commonality of Experience
Mirrors to Daily Life

On Learning
The journey to Mental Health Worker is not as straightforward as other careers. For this reason, I thought you might find my journey interesting. This is by way of validation. I was among the first tranche and therefore experienced some of the difficulties of all pioneers. I hope this is not the case for you, but as your a career is about people, it is another experience to consider and I hope will answer some of the anxieties of being an adult learner, particularly if you are not academic.

I remember being told as a teenager by a wise teacher, how experience is the best teacher. I always remembered this, though I did not realize its significance until decades later. I really value my life as a tool of learning, no matter how much I crave to be an academic loaded with degrees. I am a butterfly learner. This is good in one sense, because it means I surprise people with my broad interests. When I have a fascination, as I do mental health, I gather information from all kinds of sources, taking pleasure in finding obscure information not typically associated with the subject.

I was delighted when I started University at 52. I yearned to be a proper scientist rather than feeling an outsider, due to a lack of academic confidence. I was creative, loving writing, but was lead to believe this was not as important as science. Then I read about Einstein, deducing the theory of relativity by imagining himself riding on a sunbeam. Now I realize scientists MUST be creative, to imagine the hypothesis which precedes the experiment or research. I was enabled to link my creative ability with my analytical self.

I think I want to say, do not despair if you do not consider yourself deeply intellectual. We ALL add value because of who we are, what we have done and how we reflect upon and apply our experiences.

Why Do We Become Analytical?

I believe people from dysfunctional childhood backgrounds naturally become analytical or curious. We want to know why and what, because it is comforting and makes the world feel safer. This trait is a lifelong habit - and a good one. I've experienced episodic depressive illness since childhood. Although there were few clinical episodes, depression coloured my thinking and affected my energy levels for decades. I don't think many people, even Doctors, realize how far the effect travels across the psyche and how long lasting it is. It has far-reaching implications, including the loss of social contact which is so vital for learning hidden social rules.

My own lack of social contact was exacerbated both by depression and an autistic spectrum disorder . I was not diagnosed until my 50's but it was rather a relief, as it explained why I felt different, was considered weird and why I was singled out for bullying at school and at work. However, it was autism and a need for solitude, also a desire for recovery space, that gave me the time and energy space to develop my talents and interests.

It was common in the 1950's for childhood depression not to be recognised. My mother considered me lazy, abstruse and aloof and my peers did not accept me. I was bullied because other children tend to do this to those who are different. In fact, I was often tired, highly anxious and lonely. I did not care to share this with others, because I learned that if you share your ideas and feelings, people bully you more. This is a common experience. Years before I started working in the field, even before I knew what mental illness was, I studied people by reading mythology. This was at a very early age when most children were playing games or joining clubs. I suppose my rationale was that if I could understand what was happening in the world, I would understand how it operated:

- I would lose my fear of going mad - age 6, I heard mother saying my aunt was mad and I thought I would be too!
- I would be able to control my world
- I would understand my inner world

Later, when I started to fight depression, I noticed I could control my mood if I caught it at the right point in the cycle. The episodes gradually started to shift further apart. And I thought, hey, I wonder if other people know this - people like me? Then I knew I wanted to work in mental health, to make a difference. And, sure, it would make me feel good too. Sort of wanted and needed.

Commonality of Experience

When I came into the field as a trainee, I started talking to colleagues, trainers, patients about their life experience and realized most people have some kind of mental problem. I do not necessarily mean enduring mental illness but anything from anxiety, obsessions or tendency to moodiness.

It was a revelation and a relief. Although it seemed obvious to others, to me I was relieved I was not in a minority. This is why I am determined to share my knowledge and take the risk of revealing my inner-self by way of sharing learning, though I hope readers will respect this information.

Figure 5 Continuum 2 - Mental Health to Illness

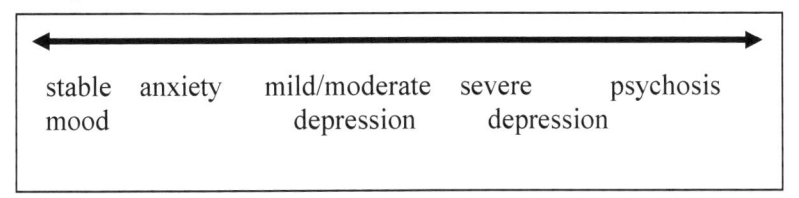

| stable mood | anxiety | mild/moderate depression | severe depression | psychosis |

When I learned about the continuum of mental illness this confirmed my thinking. Everyone has the potential to become mentally ill and everyone is anxious about something. Note I have drawn the scale in the diagram with a double-headed arrow. This is to demonstrate that even at the far end there is a way to stability.

I began to wonder where my peculiar experiences were coming from (that is to say, psychotic experiences). Surely if I no longer regarded myself as an isolated subspecies but a normal human, what were these disturbances to perception about? I began to read avidly about human experience, watch serious documentaries, order obscure books from the library (how patient those librarians were!) and scan internet sites. I was fascinated by world religion, mythology, archaeology, anthropology, serious crime and detection. I wanted to understand the mind. Never having been a social animal, this was difficult. How could I observe people, though not be in close quarters with them? There were many answers:

- books
- the Internet - specialist interest groups
- e-newsletters and journals
- special interest groups
- mythology and ethnographic study
- watching colleagues interact
- café watching (wearing dark glasses in the summer to hide myself better)

From my people-watching, it became clear the spectrum of what passes for normal is wide-ranging. Most people consider themselves 'normal' yet at the same time they want to be considered unique. What a conundrum.

Mirrors to Daily Life

I started to consider, in 2002, how the symptoms of mental illness resemble sequences in daily life. That is why, although mental illness can be frightening, it is also humanising. I would like to demonstrate this by looking at parallel experiences. That is not to say I am taking away the enormity and suffering of mental illness – this is also fact; but the more we understand it in terms of the everyday, the less stigma will attach itself to these conditions. Take a look at the diagram on the next page. It is not an easy thing to do and I will refine the process as I update these books.

See if you can add your own, after talking to patients.

Key Learning
- mental health is unlike other fields, in that it heavily relies on understanding human experience
- consider why you entered the field, your expectations, dreams, what you knew before, what you have learned about yourself and others
- consider where you fall, on the continuum line. Monitor yourself, out of interest.
- people watching is an under estimated skill in mental health
- consider the experiences patients bring to you, in terms of your own experience. Are there parallels? Try to keep a journal and make notes, without of course breaching confidentiality.

Figure 6 Parallel Experience

Symptom	Experience
OCD - checking & testing	Have you left your home then had a feeling you had forgotten to lock your door or switch off the oven? Doing this once or even twice could be considered 'normal'. In Obsessive compulsive disorder [OCD] checking is continuous. Imagine the anxiety.
despair of depression	The depth of isolation during bereavement or loss of a deep love, mirror the isolation in depression.
Mania Euphoria / exhaustion	Emotional overload and exhaustion are connected with any happy event; marrying, childbirth, a cup final. Imagine going through euphoria outside your control for days or weeks. No one can cope with such emotional overload. In mania, euphoria is frightening, with thoughts and actions so rapid the mind and body become exhausted.
visual hallucination	Seeing or feeling loved ones who are dead is common after bereavement. If no one told you, it is frightening. But imagine a Doctor told you out the blue that the people you had been seeing were hallucinations? The movie, A Beautiful Mind, depicts this brilliantly.
auditory hallucination	Have you half-heard something unpleasant being said about yourself? Imagine hearing crucial voices when there's no one about. Disembodied voices are terrifying, even when they are not 'saying' obnoxious things. I've heard such voices - their onset sets my nerves jangling, because they are 'outside' myself.
psychosis - (paranoia)	Do you recall a nightmare which re-occurred when you woke and then went to sleep again? In psychoses, nightmares continue day and night until medication calms the brain chemistry.
depression	imagine hearing bad news; a death in the family or a fatal accident. Do you recall the sense of unreality, unable to take things in. This shock/inertia mirrors the helplessness and isolation of depression.
Autism	Turn the TV to full colour and sound. Try to hold a conversation. Can you makes sense of it? Then imagine a party where all your critics will be present. Do you still want to go?

DIAGNOSIS

'Our smallest actions may affect profoundly the whole lives of people who have nothing to do with us.'
Somerset Maugham, Virtue

4   PRE DIAGNOSIS: MORAL & SOCIAL ISSUES

Content
Free to Roam?
Why Mental Illness Can Be Difficult to Spot
        Dangers of Over Reacting to Symptoms
Early Stages
Action for Relatives
Hospitalising Without Sectioning
The Case History
The Impact of Diagnosis
Reasons for Non-Arrival of Patients
Danger of Making Assumptions about Diagnosis
Lack of Mental Health Education

Free to Roam?
    Many people outside the field wonder why people with serious mental illness are not always in the care of professionals, as if such people were in some invisible community prison, constantly monitored. This sort of thinking happens after a murderous attack and there are panics about public safety. People in Western society are free to more or less do what they like unless they break a law. No one can be hospitalised or imprisoned 'without just cause' and certainly not because a neighbour thinks them a nuisance or they appear to act strangely. Our laws both protect and make us vulnerable. There has to be sufficient evidence to convict a criminal or forcibly hospitalise a dangerous patient, without acting indiscriminately on innocent or eccentric persons not harming anyone, even if their behaviour is annoying. For example, one of our patients was masturbating outside his window. Though some neighbours wanted him arrested, one kindlier soul understood his loneliness and discretely chivvied him inside, before his Social Worker arrived. Not everyone is so tolerant and I don't think I would be either, having experienced a neighbour with a hysterical personality disorder banging pans and shouting at me. We have to consider all sides, and neither be evil witch or moralising sermonizer.
    The Crown Prosecution Service decides whether or not to prosecute a suspected criminal. The police must present a good case with written evidence like witness statements, alibis, confessions. Forensic scientists look for physical evidence; DNA, fibres, fingerprints. If there is enough evidence

the CPS prosecutes and the criminal is taken to court. In the case of mental illness, evidence or diagnosis is difficult to obtain because most of it is hidden in the three areas of thinking, feeling and behaviour. A Psychiatrist and his team must prove to a Tribunal that the potential patient is seriously ill and a danger to themselves or others. If the Tribunal are in agreement, the ill person becomes a patient under whatever Mental Health Act is in place. Treatment follows. Neither mental health professionals nor the Tribunal forcibly hospitalise someone if they are not ill enough to warrant such treatment, because they will be breaching human rights.

It is difficult to decide the point at which reasonable behaviour turns into something that requires police intervention. No professional worth their salary will want to have their patient sectioned, because this will seriously affect that patient's future. This is why they err on the side of caution whilst the public see only bizarre behaviour they want out of their street, no matter what the consequences.

Why Mental Illness Can Be Difficult to Spot

It is easy to see signs of mental illness when they are full blown, but these may have:
- taken months or years to manifest
- no outward sign –a suicidal person who has not shown mental anguish
- happened away from home
- happened so quickly everyone is taken by surprise
- the result of an unforeseen catastrophe

If a patient already has a diagnosis, the family should have:
- a professional on hand, even if they have to wait for an appointment.
- a comprehensive care plan, compiled during remission
- an aftercare programme of support.

These measures are to ensure no patient who needs care slips under the net; yet they continue to do so. For those who are not regular mental health service users, the problems are difficult from first awareness to diagnosis and treatment. Why is this? There are two periods of time involved in the onset of mental illness. Some take months or years to manifest. Changes can be so subtle even close family will not be aware until family life starts to break down or a serious incident happens. In some cases, onset is so fast it knocks everyone for six.

We all have days when nothing goes right and we get irritable or withdrawn; these are normal reactions to adverse situations. Teenagers are prone to dark moods and changes in character. So how does anyone recognise signs which need attention; stress, early stages of depression or

severe mental illness? It's a bit like detective work; slowly and painstakingly gathering evidence - general indicators:
1. change in behaviour not associated with specific events
2. changes for the worse in appearance, hygiene or weight
3. marked change to usual routine
4. changes in mood which are otherwise inexplicable

These are examples which might be cause for concern:

Change In Behaviour
- quiet person becomes snappy or aggressive
- confident person becomes withdrawn and tearful
- outgoing person stops socialising
- someone good at their jobs begins making mistakes

Changes in Appearance, Hygiene or Weight
- clean and tidy person becomes dishevelled
- puts on or takes off excessive amount of weight in a short time
- gait changes - confident to slouched & lack of eye contact
- clothing suddenly either drab or too colourful or bizarre with no reason

Withdrawal or Marked Change to Usual Routine
- increased social activity to excessive level
- furtive instead of open about where they are going
- withdraws or hides from people
- stops enjoying activity

Changes In Mood Which are Inexplicable
- quiet person becomes loud and vociferous
- confident person becomes sad or fearful
- calm person is aggressive or excessively anxious

These signs appear over a considerable period of time; months instead of days. Imagine how stressful this is for relatives let alone the potential patient.

Dangers of Over Reacting to Symptoms
If a relative over reacts, most likely they will be rejected and left feeling hurt or mystified. Their loved one might feel misunderstood (if there is a rational cause and they have chosen not to share it, through embarrassment, shame or fear of over burdening relatives). Rational causes vary:

- job loss, not revealed to loved ones out of shame
- sexual or intimacy problems
- bullying, structural or management or status changes
- financial problems
- diminishment –work, school, profession
- close friend with serious problems
- health issue which they don't want to worry relatives with

If a professional over-reacts, they risk:
- being rejected when the patient really does need help
- being seen by relatives as patronising
- giving the patient a false label of mental illness
- losing the trust of patient and their relatives
- losing credibility and confidence in their expertise

Watchful waiting, as the Government calls it, is the key. Relatives might visit you, perhaps having suffered months without sharing their fears. Whilst convention says the patient must ask for help, please consider THEY [the relative] are the patient at this moment.

Early Stages

Although you cannot act, you can listen and suggest to worried relatives:
1. look after their own mental health
2. unobtrusively monitor their loved one
3. keep life as normal as possible
4. don't give up pleasurable activity, socialising or routines
5. make sure they are supported by a named professional
6. offer an advance appointment, even if months ahead
7. encourage them to keep a progress plan or a journal - maintain hope
8. watch out for the crisis point and dive into action

Action for Relatives

First Stage

Relatives will know the patient better than you. They will want to help and will be able to gauge reaction. They can put themselves into their loved one's shoes to ask a rhetorical question 'what do I [patient] want from [relative]'. If the patient is not willing to talk, it might be easier indirectly
- nice card or letter
- talking during a walk or outing

All these may open channels of communication. The relative[s] need to put the onus on themselves, avoid blaming and use the term 'I' not 'you make me..' thus:
- ♥ 'I hope I haven't got this wrong, but I feel ...'
- ♥ 'forgive me if I say this because I am concerned..'
- ♥ 'I am feeling anxious that..'
- ♥ 'I really want to talk about ... because I care for you'

Trust is easily lost and it is not anyone's business to over-interfere with another's life, even a spouse or partner.

The Crisis

Monitor, watch and wait until the crisis happens. When it does, the relative or you must dive through this window of opportunity. There will be an event or situation, or moment of realization. It may be a breaking of a pent-up emotion; something heard, read or seen that triggers reaction; a sudden insight by the loved one they are not well; a critical act that triggers the need for professional intervention.

Hospitalising Without Sectioning

My personal experience is when a friend had a manic attack and I was called by her worried parents. She was very ill, wandering around the rooms with matches, then lying on the floor talking to her voices. After a couple of hours listening to her rambling, I pleaded with her, that she was not well and please could I take her to hospital. As soon as she said a faint 'yes' I took her to my car without saying anything else. No arguments, forcing or police– it was very calm. Half an hour later she was sedated, in bed on a ward. My point is, this is better than several burly police- men arriving on a doorstep and manhandling a terrified young lady who is under a delusion they are attacking her. Or, as in my case, hanging onto an exterior pipe, and believing the police were devils trying to prevent me reaching the pearly gates. Oh, how embarrassing it all is when you return to sanity, which is why it must be sensitively handled; we DO remember what happened, after.

The Case History

The first point of diagnosis or analysis, is a case history or whatever your profession chooses to call this stage (for mental health workers generally, it is a social care plan). Without this knowledge, you cannot move on to the care plan. As an example, it is no use recommending warm baths if your patient:
- ☹ does not accept they have a problem
- ☹ is unwilling to be treated

- ☹ believes you have the problem, not them (not uncommon!)
- ☹ is afraid of water

So the order of progression is:
- taking a case history
- making an analysis / diagnosis
- producing a care plan / prescribing

Incidentally, I don't think there is anything wrong with making recommendations to patients about social care, but be careful how you do it. Do not say, 'xx will work' because if it does not they will come back to haunt you. However, you could say you heard anecdotally xx might work then leave the patient to decide. That leaves ownership of the problem and solution in the patient's hands. If xx does work, they retain kudos although you might hear later, to your chagrin, their therapist was 'no use because they solved the problem themselves'! Count this a success, not a failure on your part. A case history comprises a number of elements:

- name, address, contact, family next of kin
- background to the problem e.g. when it first occurred
- what it prevents them doing or symptoms
- what is happening now
- what the patient wants (outcome)

There are also any number of statutory forms, which I am sure you will become familiar with over time. How each therapist goes about their case history and subsequent diagnosis varies and I cover these in a later chapter.

The Impact of Diagnosis

Imagine the impact on someone newly diagnosed with schizophrenia, perhaps after a particularly unpleasant experience of visual or auditory hallucinations. How do they survive the moment they are told their realities are unreal? Imagine for yourself the psychic shock. I suggest you watch the excellent movie "A Beautiful Mind" which vividly portrays this question. This movie is the moving story of mathematics genius, Professor John Nash, who after a lifelong battle with schizophrenia won a Nobel Prize for his economic theories. Very highly recommended viewing for students of mental health.

Reasons for Non-Arrival of Patients

Some potential patients do not come to attention of a professional and rarely will because:

- families tolerate odd behaviour
- abusive families create and absorb crises; even experienced Social Workers are fooled into thinking them 'normal'
- depressive illness are perceived as sadness or laziness
- mania is tolerated as high jinks by dysfunctional families
- people are cared for within their own culture/ community
- goes unobserved in those who live alone
- family shame prevents disclosure
- suicide figures are hidden because Coroners with insufficient evidence record deaths as by misadventure –to protect relatives feelings
- some illness spontaneously go into remission

In the case of seriously ill patients lacking insight or under psychoses, medication is prescribed but not taken and appointments not kept. Some families collude under the false belief the problems will go away.

Under conflicting demands of human rights versus mental health legislation everyone is in a dilemma. The police cannot arrest and detain a person because someone claims to be afraid of them or a malicious person says something untruthful or someone misreads a situation. Both medical and legal people need to be sure there is a good outcome for all; patient, relatives and the public at large.

Danger of Making Assumptions about Diagnosis

As an example, one of my early blunders when I practiced as a hypnotherapist was treating a man who came because he had lost a valuable wrist watch. I thought his presenting problems were time and disappointment. It was too many sessions before I realized he had recently been bereaved of his wife. His search was symbolic for lost time, not the watch. But do not beat yourself by what you don't know, as long as you learn from it.

Lack of Mental Health Education

The vast majority of the public have never been educated about mental illness. Imagination is the source of fear; that and scapegoating as I have already explained. Now that citizenship and health are part of the national curriculum, this problem could be better addressed in the decades to come. However, it will take longer thanks to the Government encouraging schools to discuss mental health but not insisting upon this as part of the standards. What a waste of a golden opportunity.

****

Key Learning

- many people wonder why everyone with active mental illness is constantly being monitored. This stems from sensationalist headlines about murders, often wrongly attributed to mental illness
- many reasons for potential patients not arriving for a diagnosis
- relatives and workers need to keep watchful waiting, attempting to take ill relatives to hospital with the minimum fuss and anxiety
- it is possible to persuade ill patients to hospital, but it takes time
- the first point in diagnosing is always the case history which gives the backcloth to the current episode and often suggests the treatment
- there is a huge impact on patients to being diagnosed
- we should perhaps not be surprised when patients fail to arrive
- lack of mental health education is the source of much fear and ignorance and is perhaps an area mental health workers could usefully improve on

'Davis, like many investigators, was disposed to find what he looked for.'
H G Wells, Star Begotten

5   DIAGNOSING MENTAL ILLNESS – MEDICAL MODEL

Content
Terminology: Diagnosis v Assessment
The Aim of Diagnosis
Steps For a Typical Medical Diagnosis
Cultural Factors and Diagnosis
The Diagnostic Manual [DSMIV]
MIMS

Terminology: Diagnosis v Assessment

Diagnosis is a medical term, Greek in origin, and means to distinguish. In my dictionary it is described as 'identification of disease by investigation of symptoms and history'. Diagnosis is a medical term although many alternative practitioners use the term too. Other therapists prefer to use assessment, which does not smack of drugs or surgery. Those who practice complementary medicine do not follow the medical model, so interpretations of the patient's problem are different in outlook. For example

- a doctor might diagnose phobia and treat it with medication
- an alternative practitioner might see the problem as psycho-social, spiritual or symbolic distress and treat with psychotherapy or herbs
- a psychologist might see the problem as behavioural and encourage the patient to face the phobia in stages (systematic de-sensitization).

The Aim of Diagnosis

In diagnosing, a doctor is:
- discovering how the problem affects the patient
- trying to understand the origin of the illness
- taking note of symptoms
- offering treatment to alleviate symptoms
- planning aftercare to prevent relapse

I will use the analogy of decorating a room to explain diagnosis. In DIY as in other projects, there are stages:
1. awareness something is wrong
2. sizing up the job
3. making a list of what needs to be done
4. listing the resources required

5. make sure the resources are available
6. carrying out the plan
7. check and make sure the project is successful

Decorating a room without a plan might lead to disaster. Jobs in the wrong order and having to be done again, ordering the wrong quantities of materials, selecting colours that do not match and end up unhappy, after spending a lot of money. Incorrect diagnosis leads to wrong treatment, sometimes wrong medications, distressed patient, angry relatives, lost time and embarrassment. There is no guarantee a correct diagnosis will result in a successful outcome, but there is at least a fighting chance of success.

Steps For a Typical Medical Diagnosis
Case History

A case history enables the patient to tell their story. Telling the story is as important to the patient's wellbeing as the rest of the steps and those in the talking cure therapies would consider this a vital aspect of treatment. Taking a case history does not always happen in one session as in Primary Care, but may take several appointments. The clinician is looking for:

1. the chain of events which lead to the illness
2. if the patient has had similar episodes (instances) before
3. family health history, physical and mental
4. changes in mood and/or behaviour
5. how the patient is feeling at present

These questions will enable the professional to establish:

6. where the problems might have started
7. how well the patient is able to deal with life
8. if there is a history of similar illness in the family
9. how long the illness has been affecting the patient
10. a quantifiable measure of the problem

Mental & Physical Examination

The patient might be asked to complete psychological tests (e.g. Becks Depression Inventory, an Anxiety Questionnaire) to determine their mental state. A physical examination will help narrow down the illness and its severity. For example a blood test with high levels of lithium in the blood indicates mania.

Application of Diagnosis

Once examinations are complete, the Psychiatrist is ready to apply knowledge, using DSMV or a similar manual (see below) and make an initial diagnosis. This diagnosis may change as further evidence comes to light. As well as formal training, Doctors use their life experience, for example knowledge of cultural or ethnic considerations which may affect diagnosis or treatment. Mental illness cannot be divorced from its setting and it is vital that all facets of the patient's life are taken into consideration.

Cultural Factors and Diagnosis

As an example, black youths culturally do not give eye contact, which is considered rude; people with autism do not offer eye contact – it is one of the traits of autism; in Western culture, lack of eye contact is considered rude or evasive. Some cultures accept phenomena which in Western culture would be interpreted as hallucinations or delusions:

- voodoo and witchcraft cultures
- religious ecstasies, spiritual images or speaking in tongues
- ancestors appear to the living to advise them
- spiritualists communicate with the dead

A Psychiatrist has to take cultural belief into account when trying to diagnose schizophrenia, for example. Schizophrenia remains hugely stigmatised. A patient might be wrongly diagnosed if his culture accepts spirits, dead ancestors or ghosts as real, whereas the Western Psychiatrist believes these are manifestations of psychosis. (What would give the Doctor a better clue is his patient's behaviour/attitude –e.g. fear or lack of orientation to what was happening during the interview).

The Diagnostic Manual [DSMV]

Psychiatrists use a version of The Diagnostic and Statistics Manual (DSM). This manual is a publication produced by the American Psychiatric Association and is used world-wide to aid diagnosis. The current manual is DSMV. This contains lists of criteria (conditions) for mental conditions which are currently regarded as mental illnesses. As a piece of social history, homosexuality used to appear as a mental illness but no longer does so.

DSMV contains a list of symptoms for each disorder and a range of severity. Guidelines are based on observation and research. Each condition has a set of numbers and letters called keys, allowing the clinician to gauge the severity of the condition.

MIMS

Have you ever wondered how GP's know which of many pharmaceutical preparations to choose when prescribing? They use another manual which describes not only the chemical content of each drug but also contra-indications, dosage and cost. A contra -indication shows the clinician where a drug reacts badly with another drug or a food stuff.

Mims is 'the most up-to-date prescribing information for doctors and pharmacists' according to the publishers. Haymarket Medical is a specialist publisher for the medical field. Mims is a quarterly booklet which contains all the information doctors need to make clinical decisions. MIMS is available on-line. All the drugs in Mims are licensed (a process I described in Understanding Mental Illness) not only via drug trials but a legal license issued by the Department of Health.

****

Key Learning

- Diagnosis - a Medical Term. Many alternative practitioners do not use diagnoses in the medical sense; they prefer a holistic approach; mind, body, spirit.
- Stages -case history, mental & physical examination, analysis, diagnosis (using DSMV & clinician's experience, prescribing, treatment, aftercare
- Cultural factors – must be taken into account when making mental diagnosis
- use of MIMS to prescribe medication and avoid contra-indications between medications and also foodstuffs to be avoided whilst taking the medications

> 'There is pleasure sure in being mad
> Which none but mad men know'.
> Anon

6   MAJOR MENTAL ILLNESSES - SYMPTOMS

Content
Brief Psychotic Disorder
Depressive Illness
Eating Disorders
Mania
Obsessive Compulsive Disorder (OCD)
Phobia
Schizophrenia
Model Answers for Diagnostic Exercises in final Chapter
Solitude

Let's now consider the symptoms of the major mental illnesses. The following are symptoms according to the medical model. A complementary or alternative practitioner offers different explanations which is why talking cures and alternative therapies appear in separate chapters.

I have given you a diagnostic exercise in the final chapter, one vignette for each of the diagnoses in this chapter. The answers are in the last paragraph, so don't read them until you have looked at the vignettes!

****

BRIEF PSYCHOTIC DISORDER

Symptoms:
- Hallucinations – visual / auditory
- Delusions – powerful beliefs not based on reality
- Withdrawal and isolation
- Dishevelled appearance
- Inability to care for the self

Brief Psychotic Disorder is the medical term for what is colloquially called nervous breakdown. It is not a breakdown of the nervous system but hyper-active brain chemistry, resulting in extreme [heightened] sensitivity. During psychosis, everyday perception recedes under increasing delusions and hallucinations. Life becomes highly disorganised because it is impossible to separate the everyday real world from the delusional one. In other words, the patient loses insight into the fact they are ill and that what is happening is not real. Closest to the experience of psychoses are nightmares. Imagine waking from a nightmare to find you are still in it; that person or thing is still chasing you. Imagine the horror, were you to wake and find your partner or spouse lying dead next to you – and you had killed them under a delusion they were attacking you. Next time you hear about a mentally ill murderer, remember this scenario. Such people do not kill from cold bloodedness, but under the influence of powerful delusions. The most vivid depictions of psychosis I have seen are in these movies:

- **A Beautiful Mind** - which depicts the life of mathematician John Nash. I recommend this movie to all students of mental health. Nash was an exceptional person and managed to cope with life-long schizophrenia by using his gift of analysis to challenge his visual hallucinations. Nash realizes his hallucinations never grow older. It is enough for him to retain a precarious grip on reality.

- **The Matrix** – a science fantasy where Neo ('The One') has to get inside a computer game to free mankind from the virtual reality matrix into which robots have entrapped them. Neo experiences a blur as he moves inside and outside both worlds, not knowing which is real and which is not – perhaps both are not.

Of all mental symptoms, psychosis is the most terrifying and damaging. Some do not recover. In the case of schizophrenia, psychoses can be controlled by drugs, but there is no cure. If you consider the experience of delusions, its physical symptoms are more obvious;

- disorganised speech
- withdrawal from the real world
- dishevelled appearance

Imagine the fear, isolation and loneliness; what it must be like, for a loved one to experience a partner or friend in this state. It is no wonder carers of patients with such illnesses are in danger of becoming ill themselves, which is why carers are entitled to regular mental assessments.

****

DEPRESSIVE ILLNESS

Symptoms:
> Extreme low mood, which persists
> Lack of energy and sleep disturbance
> Withdrawal and isolation

- Lack of concentration and inability for self care
- Feelings of worthlessness or guilt
- Persistent thoughts of death / actively suicidal
- Persistent pain - headache (tight band' or medically unexplained pain

The difference between sadness and depression is the difference between a cold and pneumonia. People who have not experienced depression find it hard to imagine because they associate it with having the blues or ordinary life sadness. The nearest associated life experiences are bereavement and rejection in love which share pain, isolation and sense of unreality. Depressive illness manifests physically as extreme exhaustion, a feeling of hopelessness, worthlessness and enduring isolation.

This illness difficult for loved ones to deal with and many withdraw or heartily tell the patient to pull themselves together, leaving the depressed patient feeling guilty as well as isolated and misunderstood. There is often associated physical pain which is unexplained by physical cause.

Suicidal Urges

Severe depressive illness can be lethal. Under the influence of this illness, people of all ages and backgrounds take their own lives. Remember the lonely death recently of poor Robin Williams. Rich or poor, class clown or business magnate, it makes no difference. Suicidal urges are common symptoms of severe depression as are hallucinations and delusions. Sometimes it is only a patient's lack of energy which prevents suicidal urges turning into actual suicide. The danger time comes as energy levels rise. this is often misperceived as recovery but is in fact the time for most vigilance.

Depression can lift spontaneously or persist for months or years. Recovery is erratic and slow and there may be recurrent episodes. There is no cure as such but the patient can learn to control the illness and to recognise the signs of impending illness so that they can seek early help.

****

EATING DISORDERS

Symptoms
- self-induced recurrent vomiting or purging
- restricting intake of food
- obsessed with body weight or food
- variable extreme moods
- tooth decay, menstrual cycles disrupted
- belief in being judged by appearance

Do you remember thinking you were fat as a teenager and when you were older you looked at your photos and realized you were a normal size? It's the same sort of mental trick in the minds of people with eating disorders. It is difficult for families to understand when their loved one weighs less than 6 stones and still believes they are fat. These eating disorders manifested mainly in girls but boys are now rapidly catching up.

Anorexia means restricting intake of food whereas bulimia is binge-eating followed by purging (laxatives or self-induced vomiting). There are some aspects of both in eating disorders so doctors no longer separate anorexia from bulimia. Patients are obsessed food and crave it, however, the drive not to eat or to purge are impossible to control and often frighten them. Eating-disordered patients do not receive the sympathetic approach they need in hospital because nurses misunderstand the illness and belief it is self-induced; a similar negative attitude shown to suicidal patients who end up in Accident and Emergency departments.

Force-feeding does not work long-term as patients do not learn to address their food obsession. Nagging does not help. Many patients fear their lack of control around food and want to be cured but are unable to do so alone. Clinicians find it hard to treat these patients knowing a large proportion of those admitted to hospital will die of multiple organ failure. There is a new community treatment gaining popularity, in which a small group of patients live together in a special hostel whilst being treated on a more informal basis. It is difficult to get people with eating disorders to talk about food. If clinicians do this clumsily they are liable to have patients walk out. It is useful to use indirect means such as physical observation, waiting for the patient to talk or asking the patient why they think their parent/teacher/friend is worried about them. Sometimes the subject of food is best avoided in favour of discussions about other problems.

****

MANIA

Symptoms
- Increase in energy [psychomotor agitation]
- Very talkative with rapid speech– excessively so.
- Decreased need for sleep
- Patient has an inflated opinion of their abilities
- Rapid swings of mood

Mania rarely manifests alone, although I did meet one such patient decades ago. Mania is the high manic-depressive psychosis [MDP]; mania and depression being at either end of the scale. This disorder has been given many labels over the years, including bi-polar disorder, manic depression and MDP or manic-depressive psychosis.

Figure 7 – Woman with Mania. Bethlem Hospital

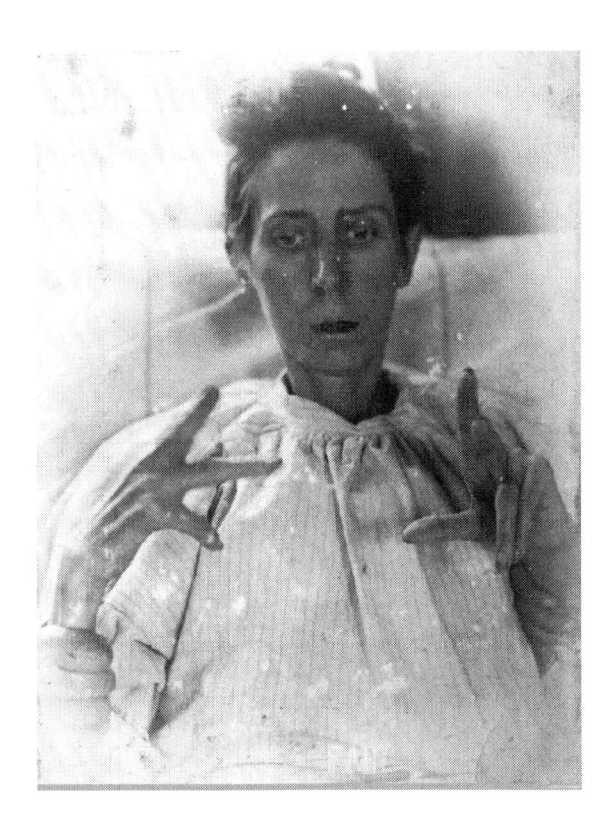

In Understanding Mental Illness, I recommended a book for trainees on MDP. Journalist Jackie Lyden wrote a biographical account of her mother's mania in Daughter of the Queen of Sheba. There are many books about mania and MDP but I found this particularly poignant as it contains a day-to-day life account of this terrible illness and the trail of destruction to family life. You may find it sobering that 20% of such patients commit suicide, an indication of their suffering.

Mania is expressed in bouts of frenzied activity and thinking. The patient is frightened about this lack of control. What it is <u>not</u> is extreme happiness. Laughing in a mirthless way is the laughter of mania. Patients in manic states may overspend, indulge in prolific sexual activity (and later be ashamed), carry out dangerous activities, act irresponsibly or irrationally to the detriment of their own and family lives. Their thoughts are irrational with an inflated belief in themselves and their ideas.

Mania cannot be controlled. The brain chemistry is over- exited and only medication can reduce it. This is one of the few mental illnesses for which medical treatment is pre-requisite. Lithium is not pleasant and after several years leads to Parkinsonism [shaking] of hands or kidney problems. It is difficult for patients with mania to continue a medication regime for many reasons:

- bad side effects
- psychological - knowing you must take a drug for the rest of your life.
- lack of insight when ill; they do not accept they are ill
- a high is powerful, like cannabis giving false illusions of power and control

****

OBSESSIVE COMPULSIVE DISORDER (OCD)

Everyone will have experienced a compulsion (urge):
- to eat or drink, even when not hungry or thirsty
- to go and do another activity
- to leave a situation because it is uncomfortable
- to make a comment, even if inappropriate

Everyone will have experienced a need to **check**:
- that you have locked the front door
- you have locked your car or bike
- you have switched off a gas or electric point
- you think you have forgotten something
- looking to the right and left before crossing a road

Everyone has **rituals** to get them through daily life:
- carrying luck charms
- actions before an event to ensure success
- religious practices or services
- football chants
- using specific numbers for the national lottery

These behaviours or rituals of checking and compulsion are normal in most contexts and are there to protect us. Imagine:

➢ if you did not check the road was clear– wham! Instant death.
➢ If you did not check the gas was off –the fire brigade hosing the remains
➢ If you did not check door was locked, possessions rifled and filth left

Obsessive compulsive disorder [OCD] comprises all these elements but to an excess. Checking is pathological when it takes over everyday life.

A common type of OCD is cleaning. When someone cleans for hours on end, scrubbing their hands raw and starting again if they miss something, this is pathological. We can say that the cleaning has become a ritual designed to ward something off – usually unpleasant thoughts or a feared event. At this point, the cleaning ceases to make sense even to the person cleaning, but they are unable to stop– it has become a compulsion. This compulsion might be persistent ideas, thoughts or images and these will only be allayed by rituals.

Mental aspects – Obsession
➢ 1: persistent idea – the house is contaminated
➢ 2: persistent thought – burglary of their home
➢ 3: persistent image – thinking about crude sexual acts

Physical aspect – Compulsion
The examples below refer to the respective numbered examples above:
➢ compulsive ritual for 1: constant hand washing
➢ compulsive ritual for 2: checking & testing of locks
➢ compulsive ritual for 3: praying to negate guilt

OCD occurs in 1.5 to 2% of the population a year. In the medical model, OCD is thought to be caused by chemical disturbances in the brain. OCD is difficult to treat and is usually subjected to medication and psychological approaches.

****

PHOBIA

Phobia is from a Greek word meaning a fear or dread. We all fear something, whether or not that fear is rational. Irrational fear is at the terror end of the scale of anxiety. Fear has ensured man's survival. If early men had not feared lions they would have been wiped out because they would not have run away. In Australia, if people did not fear spiders, there would be more deaths from poisonous spiders like the black widow. These are everyday fears:
- being out in the dark
- fear of failing
- fear of certain insects or animals
- fear of feelings like love

Phobias start as mild anxieties which spread out to areas outside the initial fear. For example mild anxiety around spiders can increase over time to phobic level, when a patient sees a drawing or crack in a pavement that resembles a spider and becomes afraid. As anxiety increases to dread, it becomes pathological and requires formal treatment. Common phobias:
- agoraphobia – fear of open spaces
- arachnaphobia – fear of spiders
- blood/infection phobia– fear of being contaminated
- claustrophobia – fear of being in a confined space
- situational phobia – fear of a certain situation e.g. flying, social phobia

Symptoms

To be diagnosed as a phobia, a condition must have lasted at least six months. Physical symptoms are the result of the hormone adrenaline which floods the body when the brain senses danger. Adrenaline causes dizziness, crushing headache, butterfly stomach, tingling, dry mouth, loosening of bowels, fast beating heart, unable to think clearly or frozen like a rabbit in car headlamps]. Mental symptoms include excessive unreasonable fear of an object and avoidance of that fear, often leading to isolation or shutting in.

Phobias have many causes, from negative encounters with the feared object in the past, to reactions to loss. Phobias are not usually treated with medication unless they are extreme in which case benzodiazepines or beta blockers can reduce symptoms of anxiety. The scale on the next page demonstrates the continuum of normal to pathological scale of fear. Fear which reaches past the cut off point [shown by a vertical line] is considered pathological and requires treatment.

Figure 8 Phobia

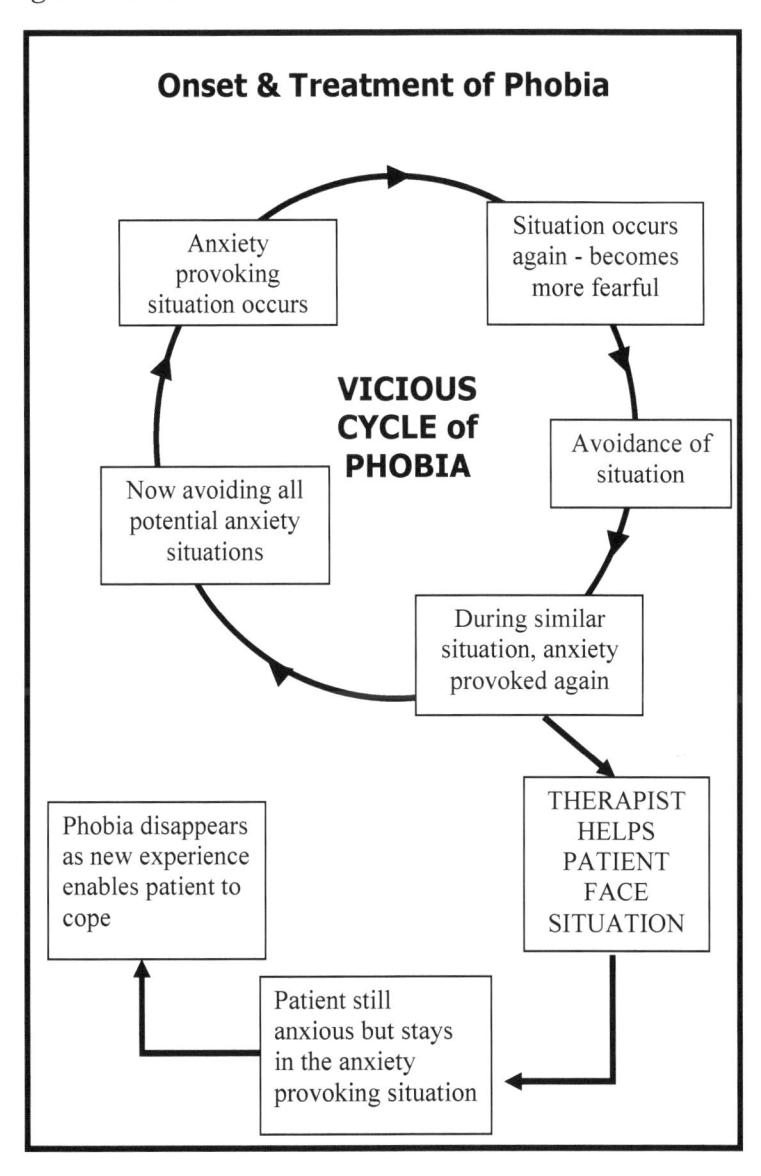

Onset & Treatment of Phobia

VICIOUS CYCLE of PHOBIA

- Anxiety provoking situation occurs
- Situation occurs again - becomes more fearful
- Avoidance of situation
- During similar situation, anxiety provoked again
- Now avoiding all potential anxiety situations

THERAPIST HELPS PATIENT FACE SITUATION

Patient still anxious but stays in the anxiety provoking situation

Phobia disappears as new experience enables patient to cope

SCHIZOPHRENIA

Schizophrenia is not easily diagnosed and some clinicians do not accept it as a distinct diagnosis. It has a cluster of symptoms that are not easily defined but understandable in terms of all or some of the following:
- fragmentation or disorganised thinking processes
- marked alterations to usual personality
- disturbances to hearing and vision – auditory and visual hallucinations
- disturbances of thinking and speech (word salad)
- loss to the normal sense of sensory input (due to above)
- loss of social status and self esteem
- gradual shunning of society – community or friendships
- marked sense of isolation
- grief or depression
- loss of sense of self as a whole person
- loss of perception of others in the same way [as above]

Schizophrenia is not split personality, however personality can be destroyed because of overwhelming and ongoing symptoms. The overarching symptoms are loss of touch with reality, fragmented sense of self-existence and inappropriate emotions leading to isolation. It affects people of all ages. It is incurable at present, although symptoms can be reduced thanks to anti psychotic medications which enable many people to live in the community.

The patient is unable to distinguish between what is really happening and what is imaginary because the hallucinations are so overwhelming they take over the sensory input. None of us can cope with massive sensory input. Many patients with schizophrenia commit suicide which is hardly surprising, given the scale of delusions and overwhelming sense of isolation.

Difficulty Explaining Schizophrenia

It is difficult to describe schizophrenia. Reading a list of symptoms does not give anything like an idea how devastating an illness it is. I have experienced psychosis therefore can find parallel experiences to explain how marked sensory perception changes your outlook, your feelings about others, your basic trust. For those who have not, look at numbers one two and three below, where I have attempted to offer parallel experiences.

Schizophrenia affects every area of what make us human; reason, trust, insight, clarity of purpose, emotions, analysis, a sense of continuity and peace of mind. Time has no meaning and there is no sense to the experiences of schizophrenia; the things that ground us in sanity – 'I am here today and doing this, tomorrow I will go here or there, this is how I will resolve that'. Imagine your world turned upside down; you don't know if it is dawn or dusk. If you want to see depictions of psychosis, look at the art of Dutch painter Hieronymus Bosch, Edvard Munch, Francisco Goya, Salvador Dali, Vincent Van Gogh, Richard Dadd and Walter Sickert.

1   Imax Cinema

The way I explained delusions and hallucinations in my last book was to refer to them in terms of an Imax 3D movie. A brief warning about Imax. Some of you might not be able to cope with the sensory experience of 3D. If you have any kind of epilepsy or sensory disturbance you should see your GP for advice before attending a screening.

Imax screens are huge, around 21 metres wide by 15 metres tall (6 doubledecker buses) with as many as 40 speakers. The curved screen and sound system surround the audience with sound and action such that you experience virtual reality. Those who regularly play 3D computer games know what it is like. During a movie, if the person sitting next to you spoke, you would be unlikely to hear, because your focus is totally on the visual and auditory input from the movie.

Imagine you are not seeing a time limited movie but that this film is with you all day, instead of the everyday world. And it is not a nice travelogue or space travel but a terrifying nightmare. It is a much enhanced type of the sensory trick of ordinary movies; daily life is suspended as we get into the story and empathise and believe in the characters. But imagine you left the cinema, and the movie continued all around you – how would you feel and react?

2   Movie – 'A Beautiful Mind'

My second example is a movie called 'A Beautiful Mind' and is the fictionalised biography of Dr John Nash, Nobel prize-winning mathematician. Nash contacted schizophrenia whilst he was at University. During his time there he was experiencing two delusional worlds; espionage and an extraordinary friendship with two hallucinatory characters, one of whom he imagined he was sharing a room with.

Astonishingly, and rarely, Nash was able to gain insight into his delusional world. He used his considerable intellect to challenge what he was experiencing, realizing his hallucinatory friends and enemies were not getting older as he and his real family aged. Nash is a remarkable man. He not only won a Nobel prize for his work but married, had a son and continued to commute daily to his former University. Sadly, the movie also depicts him being mocked by students for his behaviour and sometimes strange gait. The moviemakers cleverly merged the delusional and real life experiences of Nash to show the audience how difficult it is to separate the two - even for viewers.

3   Experiencing the Dead - in Bereavement

My third example comes from the common experience of bereaved people apparently seeing their loved one in the flesh after death. The person does not appear as a ghost or shadow but 3D as in life. In some cases, just their voice is heard but again as if in real life and talking about present experience, as if the person is still living.

These can be a very distressing experience, for those who are not expecting it and have no religious beliefs to bolster them. If you had asked any of these people if they thought such a thing possible, before being bereaved, then I doubt many would agree. However, it is a well-recorded phenomenon.

This is the manner in which some patients with schizophrenia see their delusional figures. Some see more fragmented version, as their sensory perceptions become confused and shattered by their extreme sensory experiences.

Fragmentation of Personality

Imagine for a moment life was like this all the time.

Psychiatrists describe fragmentation of the personality to be one of the traits of schizophrenia. I wonder if there is another way of looking at what are seen as individual symptoms? Perhaps the other symptoms follow on from long-term exposure to hallucinations and delusions.

Should it not be surprising that someone is unable to function as a person when their reason is unable to function due to overexposure of sensory stimuli. That in turns leads to lack of self- care, isolation, spiralling down in social terms, job loss.

- ➢ How many days could you survive such an experience?
- ➢ Can you understand why schizophrenia patients commit suicide?
- ➢ Do you understand why someone might come to falsely believe they are being attacked and defend themselves? An innocent onlooker happens to be standing nearby and is mistaken for an attacker
- ➢ Can you understand why patients are deserted; by friends and family
- ➢ Finally, do you understand why patients find it impossible to work, lose their jobs and status and end up homeless?

Next time you see a homeless person, dishevelled, wild eyed or appears drugged, consider are they mentally ill people ignored by society out of fear, misunderstanding or perhaps helplessness.

Thought Disorder and 'Word salad'

Patients may manifest word salad; a meaningless jumble of words, which patients are convinced make sense. Stroke patients sometimes have this experience too. This is an indication that brain wiring is distorted, like the white noise you hear when radio stations are not in tune.

Types of Schizophrenia
There are differences in professional views as to the different types of schizophrenia and so DSMIV is under review in this area. However, I will describe two forms I witnessed during my career.

Catatonic Schizophrenia
Now rare, catatonia stupefies the individual who sits in a semi-permanent comatose state. I remember one patient who would sit in the same chair year after year, hardly moving during the day, eating meals but never speaking. A student nurse made considerable efforts to talk to her about the past and the woman started to respond only to sink back when this nurse left and she was left to her own devices on the ward.

There were many stupefied patients sitting in hopeless silence and isolation until the advent of medication such as L-Dopa, the synthesised form of dopamine which made such a difference to their lives. Watch the movie Awakenings, the moving story of a group of long-term mental patients who were afflicted after the pandemic of influenza during the First World War.

Paranoid Schizophrenia
This type of schizophrenia is distinguished by paranoid delusion. People with this form of the illness can be dangerous if their voices direct them to kill. However shocking the acts committed as a result one has to remember this is an **illness**. Few patients are likely to commit murder but some do, which sets off the usual moral panic about all mental patients.

Confusion with Psychopathic Personality Disorder
There is an often misperceived difference between schizophrenia and psychopathic personality disorder.
- A psychopathic person is born with no sense of conscience; they are incapable of distinguishing between right and wrong [morals]
- patients with schizophrenia **do** make moral distinctions but act because they are under the influence of delusions.

Causes
No one knows the cause of schizophrenia although work is being carried out on a defective gene thought to create symptoms. There may be a combination of factors:

- University of Edinburgh is focusing on the genes DISC1 & PDE4B
- family history of the illness

- breakdown due to prolonged and extreme stress
- drug-induced schizophrenic-like symptoms

About 1% of the population is affected. Usually signs are seen during adolescence but rarely is onset in middle age.

****

COMPLETE DIAGNOSTIC EXERCISE BEFORE READING!

There is no guarantee the patient will agree to treatment or even attend an appointment for diagnosis. In earlier chapters I suggested why. Only patients sectioned under a Mental Health Act can be forcibly detained in hospital for treatment. How many case histories did you guess? Don't worry if you didn't get all or even any. To diagnose this needs not only practice but life skills and training. These exercises will help familiarise you with patterns of specific illnesses. These are not real patients but vignettes to demonstrate clusters of symptoms.

Figure 9 Answers for Diagnostic Exercises (refer final chapter)

Name	Diagnosis
Emma	Brief psychosis
Alicia	Depression
Joseph	Eating disorder
Thelma	Mania
Lesley	Obsessive compulsive disorder [OCD]
Alan	Phobia
Sandy	Schizophrenia
Soraya	Neuro Typical (mentally healthy, sane)

Were you surprised about Soraya? Perhaps you thought, as did her colleagues, she was showing signs of mental illness. Consider her culture. Soraya is torn between the culture of her parents and the Western culture in which she lives. Her parents allowed her a great deal of freedom, but in my vignette Soraya has anxieties and these are to do with cultural heritage. She is shy, a bit of a loner. I tried to portray her as the sort of girl who will not want to make waves with her parents. Her anxiety is about the boy she met in the restaurant and with whom she has fallen in love. Hence those takeaways.. Her anxieties increase, resembling symptoms of mental illness.

Let us imagine there is a good outcome and that her symptoms reduce; she has support from colleagues and is loved by her family so the prognosis is good as long as she can square things with her family. Now, if our budding Psychiatrist had questioned her and made an over-rapid diagnosis(of what?), Soraya might have had a different outcome.   I hope you can see some of the consequences raised by this vignette.

****

Solitude

Solitude is a state many wish for until they get it. There are negative and positive things about all states of being. When people choose solitude as a lifestyle they risk ostracism for being odd or eccentric. As in Soraya's case, those who choose this lifestyle can as fulfilled a life as the party animal. It does not mean a solitary life is alien nor pathological, although others find it threatening, probably bourn out of ignorance and fear. People have many reasons, positive and negative, for choosing a solitary lifestyle;

- prefer their own company
- enjoy pursuits that need reflection
- learn best through quiet study
- find creativity in the peace of aloneness
- find social situations uncomfortable or distracting
- have been abused or bullied
- sensory disorder [autism]   e.g. excess response to noise, light or colour

Equally, there are valid and pathological reasons for seeking company:

- enjoy the challenge of being in company
- learn through being with others
- find creativity in bouncing ideas off others
- afraid if they are alone
- scared of being seen as isolated
- cannot cope with thoughts and feelings when alone

Consider the solitary lifestyle of artists, writers, composers, philosophers, academics, monks and nuns. Is it pathology if such people use isolation in pursuit of art or spirituality? I think not. To end this chapter, a brief quotation from Anthony Storr's book 'Solitude';

'Perhaps the ability to distance oneself from over-involvement with others and the capacity to make a coherent pattern of one's life are important in attaining peace of mind and mental health.'

****

Key Learning
- Psychoses - look at parallel experiences e.g. a movie which depicts the experience
- Depression – an illness imbued with feelings of worthlessness and leading to existential isolation.
- Eating Disorders - very difficult to treat and need long-term input. Some say they are to do with control or avoidance.
- Mania - is nothing like happiness, joy or glee. It is uncomfortable, frightening, uncontrollable.
- OCD -obsession, compulsion, ritual all play a part in OCD.
- excessive sensory input - the brain usually filters excess input, except in mental illness or autism
- Imax 3D - a good way of experiencing virtual reality, a world which does not exist but you come to believe it does, because you are 'inside' the action. This is a way of imagining psychotic experiences.
- A Beautiful Mind' - movie which brilliantly depicts schizophrenia.
- visual hallucinations - bereavement can trigger hallucinations; seeing the deceased loved one.
- Isolation – delusions and paranoia make schizophrenia the one of the most feared mental illnesses.

Figure 10 Overview: Types of Treatment

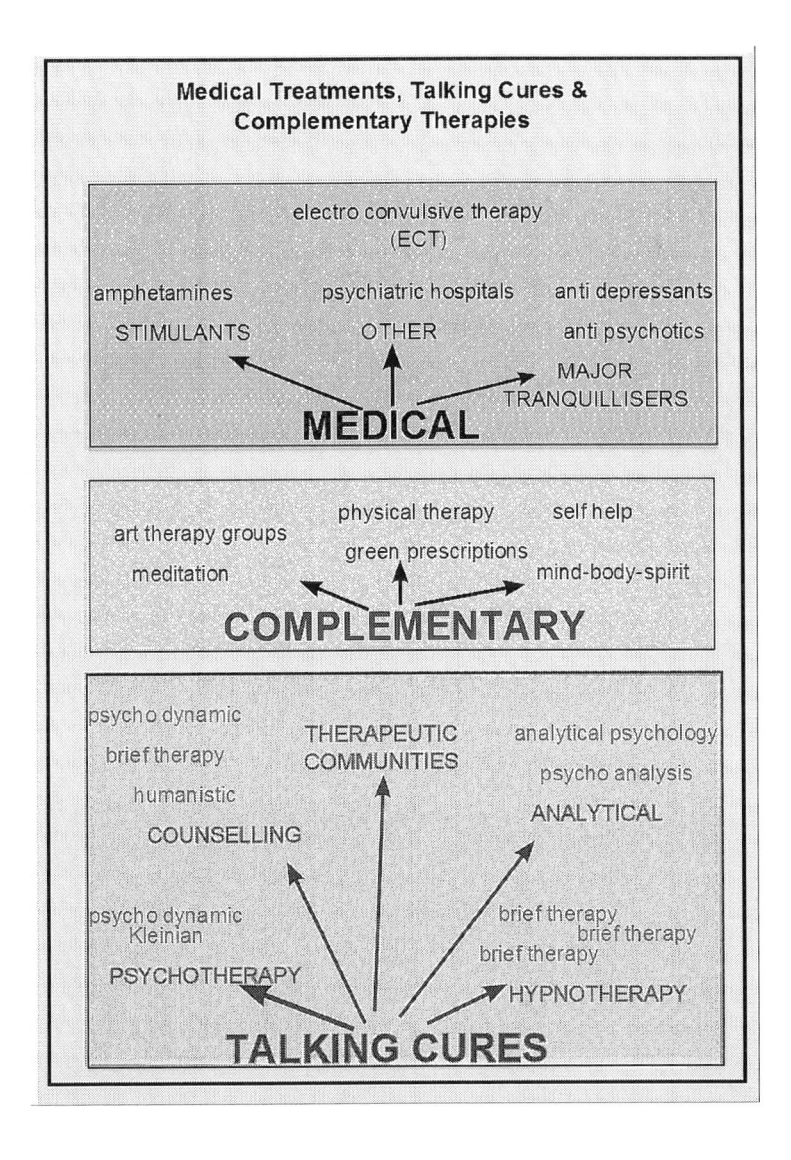

Medical Treatments, Talking Cures & Complementary Therapies

electro convulsive therapy (ECT)

amphetamines   psychiatric hospitals   anti depressants

STIMULANTS   OTHER   anti psychotics

MAJOR TRANQUILLISERS

MEDICAL

physical therapy   self help

art therapy groups

green prescriptions

meditation   mind-body-spirit

COMPLEMENTARY

psycho dynamic   THERAPEUTIC   analytical psychology

brief therapy   COMMUNITIES   psycho analysis

humanistic   ANALYTICAL

COUNSELLING

psycho dynamic   brief therapy
Kleinian   brief therapy
    brief therapy
PSYCHOTHERAPY   HYPNOTHERAPY

TALKING CURES

63

TREATMENT OF MENTAL ILLNESS

"Nearly all men die of their medicines, not of their diseases."

Moliere

7 MEDICAL & NURSING PROFESSIONALS

Content
Why Understand Other Roles?
What is a Medical Practitioner?
Can You Choose a Medical Practitioner?
How Students Study for Degrees
Confidentiality
THE MEDICAL PRACTITIONERS
   General Practitioners
   Psychiatrists
   Pharmacists
   Registered Mental Nurses

Why Understand Other Roles?

Whatever job, it is important to understand the roles of others in the field, if only to avoid inadvertently tripping on someone hallowed ground (as I have done in the past, to my cost). It is important for referral purposes; if you do not know what the rest of the staff do, how can you refer your patient, when onward referrals are required?

The medical profession is relatively new as is nursing and both are powerful bodies. I explained in my last book about my difficulties with Mental Nurses, one of whom was really obnoxious (I put this down to their anxiety about Project 2000 and changes in the profession). Similar anxieties have been experienced by new Graduate Mental Health Workers, faced with competition by Psychology Assistants. It is the Government's intention to restrict entry to mental health posts to Graduates – either other degree programmes or direct entry Graduate Mental Health Workers. Hopefully this pettiness will become a thing of the past as new entrants work their way through the system.

These situations are uncomfortable but predictable. Newcomers are feared much as silverback apes fear young offspring, whom they know will take their place at the head of the tribe one day. But try not to get mixed up in inter-professional rivalries. Those who consider themselves superior are not good teachers, and are best avoided.

What is a Medical Practitioner?

A medical practitioner is a clinician trained in medicine. These clinicians treat mental illness by prescribing drugs to re-balance brain chemistry (increase or decrease, according to the nature of the illness). Medical practitioners include Doctors and Psychiatrists. Nurses are generally grouped with medical practitioners (because they dispense pills). Medical clinicians work in hospitals, clinics, community teams and, more rarely, in private practice.

Can You Choose a Medical Practitioner?
You can choose which GP you see although in practice you might see different staff each time. Longer-serving practitioners obviously have more experience, extensive clinical connections and a lot of specialist knowledge. If unsatisfied with your GP, you can request a move to another surgery. This choice has come about because of Government policy. However, you cannot choose a Psychiatrist, Counsellor or Psychotherapist. Anyone referred to a Community Mental Health Team (CMHT) is allocated the practitioner with most space on their caseload.

For those who can afford private health care the world is their oyster and there is considerable choice, as increasingly professionals are choosing to practice privately. At this point I will not add the old joke about lawyers and teachers being professionals but doctors practising on patients as it has no place in an informative book like this. On we go then.

I'll explain first of all how a student is awarded a Degree. This applies to any Degree, not only Mental Health.

How Students Study for Degrees
Universities have various grades of student:
- Degree - the basic degree usually takes 3 years
- Honours Degree – an extra year [4 years]
- Masters degree [MSc] - a further year [5 years]
- Doctorate [PhD] - 1 to 2 research years, after a degree
- Professor – experts who teach in their field

Students are taught in classrooms or lecture theatres until they reach ordinary Degree or Masters level but after that they advance by researching or reading their subject (the terms study, reading and research are virtually interchangeable). In order to gain higher degrees, students study in their field of practice or else do research in Universities, laboratories or specialist companies.

Students read many specialist papers and books in order to gain information to conduct their first piece of research. There are indexes in Universities, like Google, where they can look up key words in their study, and will then be presented with a list of papers to choose from. This part of their research can take months.

Before they begin the research, they must apply to a special Ethics committee for approval of the methods they intend to use. This ensures no one will be hurt physically or psychologically during an experiment or piece of research. After approval, the research is carried out, with the student making careful notes. When it is completed, they are ready to make conclusions and findings, so the research can be taken forward by others. this chain of study and research stretches back to the very beginning of the history of Universities, linking all research on a firm foundation of prior studies. On completion of their first piece of research, students publish findings in a document called a dissertation. A dissertation contains:

- details of the study selected
- what the researcher hopes to learn from this study
- how they conducted the study [methodology]
- details of the research or experiment [research]
- what they found [results]
- analyses of the findings [analysis]
- how things changed as a result of the study [synthesis]
- conclusions about the study [findings]

This dissertation is presented to Examiners for marking. If the dissertation is approved, the student is awarded a degree.

As a student you are expected to do other things (apart from study) which include joking, drinking, taking part in rags (fund raising events), sport, getting in debt, worrying, living in tiny accommodation, listening to loud music, running up library fines, losing your memory stick, falling in love with your professor, falling out with friends, feeling isolated, wanting to be alone, eating out of tins, having grandiose ideas about the future. No wonder they are exhausted by year four. Sadly, none of these experiences lead to qualifications except being useful as talking points in later life.

Confidentiality

What confidentiality does not mean, as some people think, is having access to juicy gossip. Nor does it mean gossiping in the staff canteen, on the grounds they are all professionals and will not repeat it. They are not, they do and it can create havoc. Confidentiality means that a professional may not disclose personal detail about a patient to anyone, whether to a colleague, organization, legal person or relative. all records must be kept in secure places and access is restricted to certain staff.

However this has to be tempered within large organisations such as the NHS or even agencies. Confidentiality can be fuzzy. Some say is it not possible to give 100% because they must discuss patients with colleagues; but where this does happen and how much material needs to be disclosed?

Patient notes are kept centrally in the NHS and people fear their employers gaining access to this information. This is a thorny issue. I've had confidentiality about my life broken and I was angry, so I have experienced this from both sides. Apparently, trying to access unauthorized records is now a sackable offence for NHS staff.

The public are protected by law. The relevant acts are, the Data Protection, Freedom of Information and Human Rights Acts. However, professionals have cunning ways of getting around this. Do be careful what you reveal about patients. The best test is, if would you want such information spread AND might it cause danger or trouble if it is, or is not, passed on.

THE MEDICAL PRACTITIONERS
General Practitioners

General Practitioner training is divided between study, examinations and on-the-job training in hospitals, roughly 7 years worth (much being on placement not in medical school). It is not that Doctors are slow learners but they attend many placements, roughly half a year in University and the rest of the time on placement. Competition for Medical School is high and students have to achieve good science grades to be accepted onto the MBBS Doctorate courses. The term Doctor refers to the level of Degree which is awarded after passing the examinations at Doctorate level.

Your General Practitioner (GP) will have passed his degree as Doctor of Medicine (MD). The word doctor is sometimes used colloquially– e.g. 'I went to see a Doctor the other day' (compared with 'I went to see a plumber') but the correct term is General Practitioner. They need to take further training to become a Psychiatrist (6 months more) or a Consultant grade (3 – 5 more years).

Patients refer themselves to GP's for physical and mental illnesses. If a GP needs expert advice on a field like psychiatry, they will refer on to a specialist. Specialists do not see patients without a GP referral. There are specialists in all areas, for example:

- heart (cardiology)
- women's problems (gynaecology)
- mental health (psychiatry)

GP's retain clinical responsibility for patients which mean they are legally responsible for patients' well-being, even if the patients are referred on to specialists. You may notice a Doctor uses the term patient whereas other practitioners use the terms consumer, client, service user or user. These are just fashions of protocol in the same way that surgeons take the honorary title of Mr rather than Dr.

****

Psychiatrists

Psychiatrists take a degree in General Medicine then spend a year in General Practice and 6 months training in psychiatric medicine. This takes them to Junior Psychiatrist level. Five years after qualifying, juniors can apply for Consultant grade posts. Psychiatrists treat major mental illness with drugs. They administer Electro-Convulsive Therapy (ECT) where this is practised. (You may remember I said NICE severely restricted the use of ECT). Some psychiatrists take training in psychotherapy or psychoanalysis. Psychiatrists might choose to specialize in other subjects by private research or further study; these courses are called professional development.

Patient sessions with a psychiatrist last from 10 - 20 minutes, or up to an hour if they are offering a talking therapy. It is interesting that in America it is socially acceptable to visit a Psychiatrist. Psychiatric treatment (mind servicing, if you like) is seen as no worse than having your car serviced. In the UK there is still stigma but hopefully attitudes will change over time.

In the USA, health care is paid through insurance rather than indirectly via national insurance. I wonder if paying for a service has to do with the lack of stigma because services for poor people generally have stigma attached, for example benefits, social housing, charity shops.

****

Pharmacists

Pharmacists are scientists who specialize in preparing and dispensing of medicines (drugs or medications). They work in many settings:
- research laboratories - developing drugs
- hospitals, clinics and GP surgeries
- pharmacies, chemist shops or even supermarkets

Pharmacy as a science dates back to the early nineteenth century when practitioners were known by the quaint sounding names Apothecary, Druggist or Chymist. Potential students need high grade passes in science subjects such as chemistry and physics. They take a four-year Master of Pharmacy honours degree course and a one-year post graduate practical training within a pharmacy. Among the subjects they study are:
- physical properties of chemicals
- chemistry of pharmaceuticals [drugs]
- reaction of pharmaceuticals in the human body
- how to measure drug dosage

Pharmacist Subscribing

Since I last updated this book the happy news is that Pharmacists who have taken supplementary training may now prescribe. There are two grades of Pharmacist prescriber:
- **Supplementary prescriber** - with a medical practitioner e.g. GP
- **Independent prescriber** –pharmacist makes the patient assessment

Other grades of professionals able to prescribe since April 2005 are:
- chiropodists/podiatrists
- physiotherapists
- radiographers

Pharmacists can override a GP prescription if they believe the GP has prescribed incorrectly or a drug incompatible with other drugs (contra-indication). Pharmacists advise customers on over-the-counter (without prescription) medications. Some pharmacists prepare drugs from basic chemicals rather than those packaged by pharmaceutical companies.

****

Registered Mental Nurses

Mental Nurses take a 4-year degree course, working on-the-job in psychiatric settings (work experience). Their tasks are to monitor patients with serious mental illness, carry out rehabilitation work and administer medication through injection. Patients with neurotic (emotional) illnesses are generally seen by Psychologists, Counsellors or Therapists although some nurses undertake additional training in one of the talking therapies.

Consultant Nurses (highly experienced nurses) can prescribe psychiatric drugs without supervision by Psychiatrists if they have taken supplementary training. Mental Nurses work in community mental health teams (CMHT) attached to a Psychiatric Hospital or sometimes in Primary Care (GP Surgery). They see patients in a variety of venues:
- patients own home
- GP Surgery
- psychiatric hospital outpatient department

Mental Nurses give depot injections to patients who need long term medication. A depot is an injection in the buttocks or back of the hand. This administration:
- dissipates medication into body over a period of weeks or months
- lessens the need to take pills or have daily injections
- alleviates needle pain as less injections are required

****

Key Learning
- Professional rivalry –When Mental Health Degrees are base training for all workers, this will fade out
- Confidentiality - be careful what you say about patients, keep records secure. Do not be tempted into gossip. It is dangerous to your career.
- Psychiatrists - Doctors who undertake psychiatric training. Treat under medical model, using drugs and ECT, sometimes talking therapies too.
- Pharmacists - scientists trained in the nature, use and application of drugs. They are more qualified than GP's in the area of medication.

"Care more particularly for the individual patient than for the special features of the disease." William Osler, 17th Century Doctor

8   NON MEDICAL PROFESSIONALS

Content
Qualities of Therapists
Who Are the Best Therapists?
Occupational Therapist (OT)
Rehabilitation Worker (Rehab.)
Social Workers
Hypno-Psychotherapists
Psycho Analysts
Analytical Psychologist
Psychotherapist
Clinical Psychologists
Counsellors
Evidence-Based Care

A therapist is someone who gives curative treatment. It could be argued the term only applies to medically trained people but I am using it to describe anyone who is paid as a professional to:
- provide treatment for mental illness
- encourage personal development

Qualities of Therapists
A good therapist will have a variety of personal qualities and characteristics; tolerance, intelligence, well read and keep up-to-date with research. They will be ethical and understanding. They need to be resilient so they do not burn out by getting over-involved in client's problems. Are they paragons of virtue? No. Therapists are normal people, subject to normal human behaviours and reacting in much the same way to stress. Don't expect a Therapist, Counsellor or Psychiatrist to be in their role 24/7/365 or you will be disappointed. Therapists are the same as everyone else. It's what they do after that makes the difference.

Therapy is not about tea and sympathy. I have a pet theory that all good therapists had difficult lives. Like any guide, they are familiar with the territory over which their patients travel. However, they realize their patient is not going to have the same experience; that is the difference. Therapists will not be embittered, cynical or angry for too long. On recovery from such events they will learn from their experience and want to help others rather than seek revenge. So let me ask you the question:

Who Are the Best Therapists?

Imagine taking a precious car to a garage. The mechanic servicing has excellent theoretical training but has repaired few cars and doesn't drive. The young trainee in the same garage is still in training but has taken engines to pieces, re-built and serviced cars. He runs his own old banger which he services himself. To whom would you entrust hard-earned cash?

- Therapists who successfully worked through a series of life problems make excellent therapists
- Those with existing worries (99%) who have awareness (insight) and do not contaminate patient work with their own worries are effective as long as they have supervision and take therapy
- Therapists who have problems and do not know it are dangerous
- Therapists who project problems on patients or colleagues come into the forensic class (e.g. Harold Shipman)

Does your gut feeling tell you to trust this person? Then you are probably right.

****

Occupational Therapist (OT)

Occupational Therapists assess physical and psychiatric conditions and also patients with dual diagnosis. The therapy they use is known as purposeful activity, whether that be mental or physical exercises, designed to help patients undertake paid work or find suitable leisure activity.

Physically disabled patients are assessed for practical aids to overcome daily living problems; from simple actions such as opening tins of food to the more complex activities of bathing or mobility. These are things which mobile people take for granted but which can make a huge difference to these patients self esteem and participation in life.

OT's can offer practical guidance like assisting with the completion of housing or benefit forms which can be daunting to patients crippled by mental illness, physical conditions or extreme pain. OT's patients become as independent as possible within their level of capability.

Occupational Therapy is either a 3 year degree taken at a University or an in-service 4 year course, where applicants start out on unqualified grades as support workers.

OT's are not medically trained and don't either diagnose or administer medications. The role has overlaps with Social Worker, Rehabilitation Therapist and Mental Health Worker.

****

Rehabilitation Worker (Rehab.)

Rehabilitation Worker is not a widely known in the UK, being better known in the United States where Rehabs. have professional status. When I worked in this role we were on unqualified Social Worker scales, even after several years experience. Rehabs. were given patients who did not readily fall into other disciplines, mainly enduring mentally ill patients who were visited in the community. Rehabs. were the mainstay for first tranche of mental patients moving into the community in the 1990's. Proper assessment, social skills training, anxiety management and life enhancing skills enabled patients with major mental illness to live full lives in the community. I used, by dint of my private practice, qualifications and experience, to additionally assess and counsel patients from Primary Care with depressive illness and other affective disorders, but this caused such a furore I was prevented from doing this after complaints from some Mental Nurses. An example of how anxiety about role boundaries can create havoc if not managed properly. Rehab applicants were chosen for maturity, common sense and life experience. I believe there is now an NVQ in Rehabilitation available to this grade of worker, but believe the role will be subsumed by the new Mental Health Workers.

****

Social Workers

Social work trainees are 22 years of age or above with some experience of working in the field. They are selected from mature applicants as they are dealing with social problems which necessitate prior life experience. This is why the age limit is set higher than for many other professions. Social work training covers social policy, welfare and mental health law with optional short courses in basic counselling, psychology or specialist areas like learning disability. Trainees spend a proportion of their training working in-the-field (on-the-job). A degree (DipSW) in Social Work takes four years to complete. Further training to Approved Social Worker (ASW) level entitles the holder to assist in sectioning patients under the Mental Health Bill.

Social Workers work in the community, helping patients with relationship, housing or financial problems. Their main role is to monitor long term (chronic) mentally ill patients, ensuring medication is available and monitoring its use. There are two main branches from which new students can select; adult care or children and families.

There is stigma around Social Workers stemming from an old-fashioned view that they visit only working class patients. This is far from the truth. They have also been perceived as interfering in family life, particularly those who specialize in children and family work, where there are delicate boundaries between child safety and parental rights. They have also been seen as handy scapegoats for bad managers, particularly when cases have gone wrong;. Maria Colwell, Mary Bell and other infamous cases.

****

Hypno-Psychotherapists

Hypno-Psychotherapists work in private practice. Hypno-Psychotherapists are found under the umbrella organization the United

Kingdom Conference for Psychotherapy (UKCP). Basic training is around 4 years, longer than previously as the discipline has been extended to include psychological subjects, now it is integrated within UKCP.

Courses for Hypno-Psychotherapists are post-graduate level for trainees 18 years or over who have broad life experience and/or qualifications in mental health. Courses are often held at weekends to enable those who work during the week to attend. Hypno-Psychotherapists utilize unconscious processes in patients, the natural state of altered awareness known as hypnosis, deep relaxation or inward focus. In this relaxed state the conscious mind does not throw up barriers (resistance). It is easier to give an example:

> There are payoffs for staying as you are. For example, a person lacking confidence stays at home where it is safe. On becoming confident they must accept responsibility for failure and embarrassment, as well as success. But the payoff of becoming confident is sometimes overridden by fear of failing – so conscious mind 'resists' by retaining lack of confidence and staying home. This does not apply to conditions like autism, where need to withdraw is part of the pathology and cannot be altered.

The process of hypnosis is a small part of what these practitioners do and has been misunderstood. Hypnosis has been considered with awe or ridiculed. The field is gaining respect due to:
1. Nurses training in hypnotic techniques in anti-smoking clinics
2. the work of Magician / Hypo-Psychotherapist Paul McKenna who demonstrates through his stage and clinical work that the process works
3. entry of this discipline into full membership of the United Kingdom Conference for Psychotherapy

Hypno-Psychotherapists work in different ways. Some use hypnotic states to help clients break negative links with the past and re-discover problem-solving skills. Other practitioners use solutions focused (brief therapy) models to facilitate change – after the model set up by Dr Milton Erickson (American Psychiatrist). This therapy is beneficial for time-limited problems, mild to moderate depression, personal development., phobias, smoking cessation, social and relationship problems. The solution focused model (SFT) is clinically proven and approved by the National Institute for Clinical Excellence (NICE) for use in Primary Care.

****

Psycho Analysts

Psycho Analysts (followers of Sigmund Freud) are few in number and have long waiting lists. There is only a tiny amount of psychoanalysis available on the NHS because it is expensive. An analyst's training starts with their own analysis by a qualified practitioner. At this stage they hold the quaint title Analysand. An experienced analyst might spend 10 years in therapy (Analysand) before taking their formal training. Training and therapy are undertaken at their own expense so psycho analysis is elitist.

Private patients who see analysts need to have the capacity for insight, so it does not suit everyone. As analysis is expensive and time-consuming, patients need to have enough income to sustain the number of sessions; 2 to 4 a week with each lasting 45 minutes (therapeutic hour).

Before psychiatric medication in the 1950's, analysis was commonly used for patients with mania and schizophrenia. Years ago, I meet a lady who had been treated for mania and still bemoaned the death of her analyst. She had to endure a lifetime of anti-manic medication which resulted in Parkinsonism for the remainder of her life.

****

Analytical Psychologist

Analytical Psychologists follow the teaching of Carl Jung. Analytical psychology is concerned with development of personality through a process Jung termed individuation. This takes place around mid life, when we begin to look back. Through individuation people become rounded personalities and live life to its utmost capacity.

Jung believed mankind had neglected the spiritual dimension which he felt essential to becoming a whole person. This holistic view is held by all complementary practitioners who treat mind, body and spirit.

Jungian Analysts have a variety of tools at their disposal:
- dream analysis
- exploration of archetypes (aspects of personality)
- analyzing the transference

As adults, we react to certain people in the same way we reacted to similar characteristics in certain children. This is called transference. Jung helped patients to understand why they reacted in this way and with the awareness came healing. Jung also taught patients to recognise their own archetypes and integrate them within the personality. Analytical therapy is suitable for existential (life) problems such as relationships and emotional (neurotic) disorders as well as personal development for its own sake.

****

Psychotherapist

Schools of psychotherapy offer the tools (mental processes) to help people improve happiness and gain peace of mind. Psyche is Greek for mind, so think of it as therapy for the mind. Training for psychotherapy of all schools is a minimum of 4 years. This includes training, personal therapy, supervision and practice with clients. Psychotherapy is not a career for those unwilling to look deeply into their own minds. Psychotherapists must gain insight into their own personality, whether through personal therapy, co-counselling (two professionals working together) or self reflection.

Psychotherapy can work well for people with early life trauma, a process which is emotionally painful yet ultimately transformative. Analytical styles are not recommended during depression or bereavement. Clients have more autonomy than in other therapies, particularly analytical styles, for their own healing.

****

Clinical Psychologists

Psychologists take a 4 year Honours Degree in Psychology with specialist training to work in clinical (medical) settings. Psychology is a science degree based on experiment and animal research. Psychologists publish papers on mental and social issues. In clinical settings they work alongside Psychiatrists but do not necessary hold to the medical model.

Psychology is about patterns and standards; personality types and behaviours. Psychologists are looking for rational rather than esoteric qualities. It is focussed on helping patients recognise and change faulty behavioural patterns, rather than in encouraging individuality as in psychotherapy. Psychologists specialize in education, forensic (criminal) work, sports psychology or experimental animal research. Research Psychologists sometimes do not work with patients but specialise in laboratory animal experiments, looking for behaviour patterns.

Cognitive behavioural therapy (CBT) is 'flavour of the month' among Psychologists and NICE. CBT is about challenging negative behaviours. Patients complete diaries and progress sheets as part of therapy, which some might find tedious.

Clients with dual diagnosis mental illness (e.g. alcoholism and depression), major mental illness or long standing problems respond to psychological methods. Patients are seen weekly and need sufficient motivation to complete the tasks set by their Psychologist.

****

Counsellors

The term counselling is synonymous with psychotherapy. A potential Counsellor must prove he/she has resilience to deal with distressed people without becoming distressed. They can be creative in approach and accept whatever clients bring with compassion. People who are dogmatic (have strong views or alliances with causes) do not make good counsellors. All counsellors have supervision and some undertake regular personal therapy.

Counselling is no longer commonly in Primary Care as the roles have been taken over by stepped therapy training model, within Mental Health Trust teams. There are still charitable counselling organisations all of whom ask a fee although these are on sliding scales for less-well-off clients. Counsellors work in private practice too. Like Psycho Analysts, private counsellors pay for their training, supervision and therapy.

Types of clients vary from existential (bereavement, relationships), mental illness such as depression or the affective (emotional) disorders. Patients may ask for help with time limited life problems. All of these respond well to counselling. Supportive counselling may be offered to patients with major mental illness during crisis periods; that is, counselling which does not attempt to extract the root of the problem but offers emotional support.

Evidence-Based Care

The field of mental health is undergoing huge change. Although there is a general move towards evidence-based health care there is still little funding for research. Medications must be regulated because they are potentially life threatening, whereas if a therapy does not work there is no terminal damage. Until this happens, much of complementary therapy is at a huge disadvantage. But many of these have been proved to anecdotally work. Dr Kathy Sykes has shown how the therapeutic relationship (between therapist and patient) is a huge factor in healing and she has carried out interesting research on how pain centres reduce when certain complementary healings are applied. This is a very interesting area of development and worth watching.

****

Key Learning

- Experience v Training – mental health workers are life experienced and therefore need less training than young undergraduates who may have gone from school to University.
- Overlap - many therapies overlap. Boundaries can cause rivalries. This dissipates as roles are clarified over time.
- Evidence Base - there is insufficient funding to research therapies that often work anecdotally. Professor Kathy Sykes has proved these are worth investigation.

****

> 'The belief, the self-confidence, perhaps also the devotion with which the analyst does his work are far more important... than .. old traumata'
>
> C G Jung

9   TALKING CURES

Content
Behavioural Therapy [Systematic De-sensitisation]
Cognitive Behavioural Therapy [CBT]
Counselling, Psychotherapy & Psychology
Talking Cures
Modelling
Schools of Thought
Theoretical Stances
Analytical Psychology
Gestalt
Encounter Groups
Rogerian or Client-Centred Therapy
Hypno-Psychotherapy
Milton Erickson & Solution-Based (Brief) Therapy
Psychology
Reichian Therapy
Family Work

This section is about the talking therapies and psychological treatments. They do not include invasive treatments (surgery, drugs or ECT) as in the medical model. some of the therapists discussed in the last chapter use talking therapies, either as sole therapy or as an adjunct to their work.

Behavioural Therapy [Systematic De-sensitisation]
Behavioural therapy is based on Pavlov's theory. Behaviourists believe it only necessary for people alter their behavioural patterns to effect change i.e. ruts we get into; reacting in certain ways to certain situations.

Behaviour therapy can be used to rid patients of habits such as phobia. In systematic de-sensitisation, the patient is gradually introduced to the object causing the problem until it resolves. They have been literally re-programmed to behave in a different way.
Example 1
Smokers will be directed to cut down on cigarettes. They may be played videos of cancer-ridden patients or given hypnotic suggestions of how clean their lungs will be after giving up.
Example 2
An agoraphobic patient will gradually increase the distance they are able to walk from their home.

Most therapists find this therapy reductive which is why cognitive behavioural therapy (recognition or insight) is more widely practiced. Behaviour therapy can be used in conjunction with medications taken to help unwanted behaviours. It is an adjunct to talking therapy and works with habits like smoking, drinking, nail biting and some sexual perversions.

Cognitive Behavioural Therapy [CBT]

Cognitive Behavioural Therapy is based on the fact there are connections between what we think, what we feel and how we subsequently behave. This is based on learning theory. Refer diagram below.

- **initial thought** arises from unconscious and is <u>not</u> under our control.
- **follow on thought** depends on conditioning i.e. what we believe true.
- How we **feel** (consider) a situation follows the conditioned thought
- How we **behave** [respond] depends on the feeling

   - initial thought – it is raining
   - follow on thought – I wanted the sun to shine today
   - feeling – frustration and discontent
   - behaviour – go back to bed

After modification, through therapeutic input or our altered thinking:
initial thought – it is raining
follow on thought – I wanted sunshine but rain will water my garden
feeling – acceptance
behaviour – continue with the day's events

After a period of adaptation to the new thinking:
initial thought – it is raining
follow on thought – good, the rain will water my garden
feeling – contentment
behaviour – choose what to do that day

By modifying a thought about a situation, you can alter the way you feel and behave. CBT therapists say, you change the effect by altering your behaviour i.e. act 'as if' the rain is good, and it alters your feelings (attitude or perception) towards the event or situation. CBT therapists ask patients to record thoughts feelings and behaviours and altered responses.

Figure 11 Cognitive Behavioural Therapy

Triangle of Insight:

thought

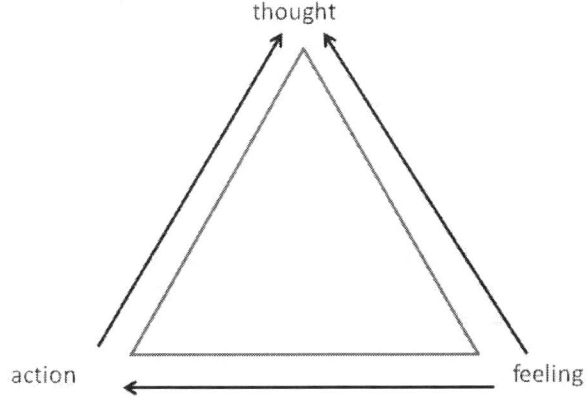

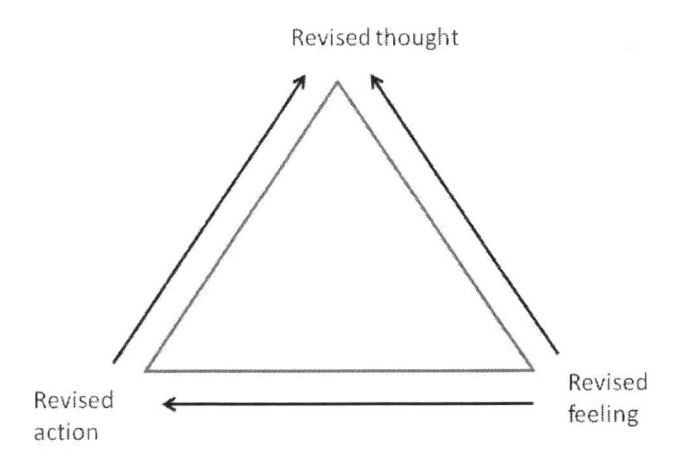

action ← feeling

Revised thought

Revised action ← Revised feeling

Uses of CBT are:
- phobias
- depression
- emotional problems
- behavioural problems

Counselling, Psychotherapy & Psychology

There are many different schools of thought for counselling and psychotherapy and many overlaps which are not even clear to some professionals. This is why I think, for the short space I have here, to describe a few of the main types and to lump counselling with psychotherapy.

The two counselling umbrella organisations each have members of from both disciplines:
- British Association for Counselling [BAC]
- United Kingdom Conference for Psychotherapy [UKCP]

Umbrellas are curious entities. I don't know if they exist in other fields but they appear to have developed a life of their own, overseeing the individual schools which make up their membership. On the good side, they offer regulation but on the negative side, they can become elitist. Those schools who cannot afford umbrella organisation fees will be squeezed out of existence as the Government tightens the noose on regulation, thus limiting training to those with large pockets. The schools did manage to self-regulate before these bodies came into power. This is another reason the punter at the end of the line, the patient with no independent means, finds it difficult to find affordable treatment, whereas there are plenty of good therapists who need to earn a living. Someone may be able to reconcile the two ends in time.

Talking Cures

Talking cure is a term coined by one of Freud's patients, Anna O., to describe how Freud cured her during hypnosis. The term is now in common use, describing all therapies using talking rather than invasive medical techniques (drugs, surgery, ECT etc.).

But how does a talking cure work? I used to explain to patients, that while we cannot move a mountain, we can move individual rocks. So over time, we can make huge changes. The patient gradually comes to recognise faulty thinking or behaviours or that there are better ways of living, or how relating differently will reap rewards and result in more happiness or peace of mind.

Modelling

Medicine targets specific areas, be it brain chemistry, neurons, or a system like breathing, heart or muscles. Doctors can pinpoint neurons and systems using brain scans, x-rays and diagrams of the human system. All these have emanated down the ages, beginning with the examination of corpses by polymaths like Leonardo da Vinci, the earliest anatomist. Early doctor-scientists drew heavily on cutting up cadavers, before the invention of CAT scans and the like made the workings of the body visible. However, dealing with the mind is more difficult.

Although the brain is a physical organ, mind is not. Mind is ephemeral. Although we assume it is cited in the brain, there is no proof. Some scientists believe memories exist in the other organs too and there is some evidence of this. Existential problems cannot be drawn in the way that anatomists draw the circulatory or the muscular system. Each mind is different, the product of its human creator, and a mass of connecting neurons which grow and change as we learn. So therapists had to find another way of explaining the workings of mind. What they came up with was modelling; diagrams which explained theories in symbolic form. The diagram of the CBT triangle earlier in the chapter is such a model.

Schools of Thought

So how did the schools of thought separate? Many people think hypnosis began with Jung and Freud but in fact it is the oldest therapy and has been used from very early times. Freud was a follower of Charcot and Breuer, two men who modernised the use of hypnosis as therapy. Freud and his disciple Jung spent their lives exploring the psyche and it is these two branches which spawned a whole line of psychotherapies (mind therapies) which include all modern schools of psychology and counselling.

What happens to continue this line is rather like our students, all studying their Degrees. A pupil of a great theorist might develop a new line of thinking, based on what they have learned. As their thinking (theories) develop, their theories expand, become more fixed through experiment and gradually are written down. This new theory will eventually attract new followers (pupils or students or devotees) and thus a new school starts. It is interesting to trace back various schools to their origins. I know this has been done in various books and websites but if you trace back the school of thought for your own school, you will get a greater sense of achievement and understanding of how the theories developed.

So your patient is inundated with choice but at the same time stymied by the cost of therapy, which is probably (for ordinary working people) about **eight times** (minimum) **the hourly rate they earn** (based on minimum wage). This is what we call progress. Perhaps you will figure out a new theory of how to reconcile this dichotomy? There's a challenge.

Let's consider some of the schools of thought. I risk the accusation of reductionism, because it is impossible to describe a school of thought to less than half a page; but there we are. If any school feels misunderstood they are welcome to offer assistance. I would like to relay this anecdote. The best teacher I had at University, when faced with puzzled looks from a student, did not say 'don't you understand?' but 'perhaps I need to explain in another way.'

Theoretical Stances
- Analytical Psychology
- Gestalt
- Rogerian or Client-Centred Therapy
- Hypno-Psychotherapy *
- Psycho-Dynamic
- Psychology [Behavioural Therapy And CBT]
- Reichian [Physical Therapy]
- Solution Focused Or Brief Therapy *

* these are linked but have many schools of their own

If you want more detail, I described a few in my book, Understanding Mental Illness. There are also many topic specific books on Amazon.

Analytical Psychology

Jung coined the term personality as a model for the amorphous mass of ideas, morals, values, beliefs, ancestral symbols (collective unconscious) which comprise our personality – or what we call the self. Personality defines who we are and how we live. This was an incredibly painstaking process which took Jung a lifetime. He began by studying world religion, spirituality and mythology. Unfortunately, he did not write his unifying theory at the end, a piece of work left to his followers.

Analytical psychologists look at a whole person rather than probing individual problems. Their aim is integration of the personality with its sub personalities (archetypes). This process peaks around mid life when the focus changes from outward doing (getting and spending) to inward thinking (reflection). Jungian Analysts call this search for the self, individuation. Through a process of maturation and insight, patients learn to recognise and avoid pitfalls, that is to deal with difficulties by using the personality, rather than having to seek help for each problem that arises. Of course, this is a far longer process and requires dedication to the process.

In order to understand the personality, the patient has to delve into unconscious mind, that is, the part of mind that is usually outside our

everyday experience. For Jung, the unconscious expressed itself most clearly through three avenues:
- the symbolism of dreams
- ancestral memories during reverie
- de ja vue (a sensation of having experienced something before)

Gestalt
'Life is not a problem to be solved but a reality to be experienced.' Kierkegaard

Gestalt follows the school of Fritz Perls, a student of psychoanalysis. It is an amalgam of psychoanalytic and humanistic principles, seeking to discover the whole person and their relationship to the world they live in, as experienced **in the now**. The above epigram neatly summarises the Gestalt perspective. Problems are not separate but are part of life experience.

Gestalt means unified, whole or the essence of something. It implies a complexity that cannot be reduced without taking something from it. In Gestalt, the environment is as important as the experiences of the patient. Gestalt therapy helps the patient into full awareness by all possible methods. Therapy is conducted in groups with group members acting as co-therapists. Thoughts, feelings, images from the past are brought into the present through asking the patient what they are experiencing in the here-and-now and exploring the resulting issues.

Encounter Groups
Encounter groups encouraged patients to relive past negative experiences whilst other members of the group made comments which supposedly changed the patient's experience of a past event. The therapy was brought into disrepute by group members using this as an opportunity to 'let out' their own dark feelings. It is easier to give an example.

A friend of mine (now deceased) was encouraged to talk about her friend's suicide. This woman had jumped to her death from a high building. My friend was horrified when one of the group started chanting 'tomato sauce', a horrific chant taken up by others, under the impression this was 'helping' her. The group leader said nothing. My friend told me how she could not wait for 'her turn', so she could extract revenge. She was usually a kind woman and this was completely out of character.

As you can understand, this practice was based on a naïve view of human nature, and easily open to abuse, particularly when the group leadership was of poor quality. It assumed too much about the 'niceness' of human nature. Although this therapy is discredited, its basis is integrated in group therapy within therapeutic communities, where there is more than one leader to control and monitor behaviours.

Rogerian or Client-Centred Therapy

Rogerian therapy is a humanistic style based on acceptance of whatever the patient brings, even if that might be shocking to the therapist. Carl Rogers was the most influential of the humanist group. It is perhaps not surprising that Rogers theoretical stance was based on unconditional positive regard. He was religious and destined for the priesthood when a chance visit to an overseas convention opened his mind to new ideas and he decided to take up psychology.

Rogers believed that humans, animals and plants alike contained the seeds of self-actualization. Mental illness to him was this same process gone astray. The task of therapy was to bring the client (Rogers' less pejorative term for patient) back to wellness, by accepting them as they were. He saw love and stability as means to re-ignite the process of actualization. Rogers called his therapy client-centred, but it is also known as Rogerian therapy. The three basic for the therapist are:

1. **Empathy** – sympathy without over involvement in patients' feelings
2. **Congruence** – being open and honest
3. **Respect –** showing consideration and understanding

Rogerian therapy conducted badly could too easily parrot or mimic the client, without appearing to understand what they brought. Sample:
Client 'I feel blue'
Therapist 'You feel blue?'

This is not only insulting but hardly likely to gain the level of empathy which Rogers envisaged. A more likely progression of dialogue is:
Client 'I feel blue'
Therapist 'So life doesn't feel good at the moment?'

Rogers wanted clients to 'launch [themselves] fully into the stream of life'. Full immersion into life was, he considered, the only way a client could self actualize. This would bring sorrows as well as joys and was not for those who were afraid of experiencing negative emotions.

Rogers legacy was a large body of humanitarian work, using his methodology to bring together warring communities across the world.

Hypno-Psychotherapy

Much derided for what outsiders saw as its apparent simplicity, hypno-psychotherapy is now respected as a therapy in its own right. The hypnotic state is a very deep form of relaxation and had been known about for centuries although not named and not understood in the modern sense of the word. Nineteenth century Doctors Breuer and Charcot used hypnosis for treating patients for hysterical paralysis. The treatment became popular and many students were curious about it and wanted to learn more. These students included the later famous Sigmund Freud and Carl Jung. It was studying hypnosis which lead to their theories of conscious and unconscious mind which were the root of all the talking therapies.

Hypno-psychotherapy students study a theory of mind, according to their school of thought, incorporating hypnosis into their therapeutic tool kit. It is still popular and comes under many guises including mindfulness, a form of relaxation therapy which is thousands of years old and was developed by Buddhist monks as a method of meditation.

Milton Erickson & Solution-Based (Brief) Therapy

Modern solution focused and brief models, including NLP, all developed from Ericksonian theory. Milton Erickson was an American Psychiatrist who encouraged followers to understand patients entering their patients' 'symbolic map of the world' (how each patient experiences their world). There are echoes of Jungian theory, but rather than explore dreams or archetypes, Erickson believed symbolism could be detected through the language used by his patients.
1. patient 1, 'I <u>feel</u> this is right. I can almost put my finger on the reason'.
2. patient 2, 'I <u>hear</u> what you are saying but there are echoes..'
3. patient 3, 'I can almost <u>see</u> them as I'm saying this.'

Of course, these are simplistic examples. Patient 1 is tapped into feelings and experiences his world through this sensory modality. Patient 2 is in auditory modality and senses the world through hearing. Patient 3 – can you guess? Erickson believed his patients could be taught to resolve problems through understanding their own 'map of the world' –
1. would be encouraged to notice <u>gut feelings</u> when faced with situations
2. would be encouraged to '<u>listen</u> to their inner voice'
3. would be encouraged to '<u>visualise</u> a different world'.

This emphasis on teaching not therapy came from Erickson's experience of successfully teaching himself to walk after being struck down with polio. Erickson was highly visual and observed his new sibling learning to walk and how visitors moved around the room. In teacher fashion, Erickson set tasks for his patients or sometimes would just talk. These therapies might appear outlandish if taken out of context but from the patient's point of view, they make utter sense. Consider these examples:
- a couple were desperate to have a child and were distraught each time they were unsuccessful. They overcame bedtime anxiety by being directed to 'fuck for fun.' Forgetting about procreation for several months in favour of fun sex, nature took its course.
- a market gardener was depressed and had given up. Erickson did not talk about depression but sent the man into a semi-hypnotic state by talking at length about plants, growth and sunlight. The gardener began to remember watching things grow and how he had nurtured them, of

how seeds come out of dying plants to continue the cycle. The gardener realized his part in this scheme and this gave him renewed hope.

Erickson did not say, use these methods for every sexually dysfunctional couple or depressed gardener but many therapists mistakenly copied Erickson parrot fashion, rather than listening to patients and this put his methods out of favour. But in the 21st century, the brief therapy methods he spawned were researched by NICE and found to be effective.

Psychology

The pioneers of psychological thinking were Freud and Jung whose work I have attempted to explain. Psychology is the study of behaviour. Research Psychologists carry out experiments on animals, such as Pavlov's work, to learn more about behaviour in humans. They draw heavily on modelling to explain theories, for example the CBT model described in this book. Some psychologists never come into contact with patients.

For further information, read the section on cognitive behavioural therapy.

Reichian Therapy

Wilhelm Reich was initially a follower of Freud and the psycho-analytic model. However, he felt the effect of the psyche on the physical body (Freud's libido theory) had not been sufficiently explored and this became his focus. Reich believed that problems in the psyche lead to physical armouring, whereby muscles become tightened and locked. His therapy comprised of physical exercises, aimed at releasing tension and thereby releasing psychic and sexual tensions at the same time. Part of his experiments were on a mysterious energy he called orgone which had two types – orgone (positive and energy producing) and DOR or deadly orgone radiation. He developed an orgone accumulator, which was a shielded box in which his patients sat to cure them of mental illness and relieve them of sexual and physical tensions. This has overtones of therapies used in Bethlem Hospital in earlier centuries. Reich's radical beliefs brought him into conflict with the authorities and he was imprisoned for breaking an injunction imposed on selling his accumulators. His books were burned by the authorities and he died in prison of a heart attack. Reichian theory of armouring was successfully taken forward in modern sex therapy.

Family Work

Mental health workers routinely work with families of patients with schizophrenia, to try to prevent trauma and disruption to family life. This is an adjunct to work with the patient. Many families find it hard to cope with relative's mood changes and tendency to withdraw, which is too easily misinterpreted as rejection. Patients do not always recognise when they are ill and refuse medication, so they become ill more often than they should. Lack of patient compliance with taking prescribed medication can lead to family breakdown, as the patient's symptoms worsen. This is distressful for everyone.

Family workers encourage the regular taking of medication and help the patient prepare a care plan. This is a kind of advance directive made when the patient is well, with directions for how they want to be treated when ill. Patients are encouraged to live a healthy, productive lifestyle which takes into account their illness. Care plans are comprehensive and creative. a care plan might include

- a patient's list of their signs of oncoming illness
- what they find helpful
- how they do not want to be treated (being just as important).

****

Key Learning

- Cognitive Behavioural Therapy – the triangle of Insight is how patients learn to recognise the links between thinking, feeling and behaviour; and how any modified by changing the others.
- Modelling - modelling is making theoretical models for psychological concepts, enabling us to learn in symbolic form how the mind works.
- Jung - Jung's life work was study of the personality. A Jungian Analyst's work is helping patients towards individuation, integration of personality.
- Gestalt - the whole is more than the sum of parts
- Rogerian Therapy - client-centred is a humanistic therapy. Rogers said patients must be totally accepted, whatever they bring to therapy.
- Solution & Brief Therapies - based on problem solving and educational methods, rather than psychoanalysis.
- Psychology - the study of behaviour. Psychologists use modelling to extract theories by studying unusual (pathological) behaviour.
- Reichian Therapy - a combination of thinking which links blocked libido to muscular armouring in the body.
- Family Work - seeking measures to combat repeat episodes of enduring mental illnesses, using a whole family approach.

> "Do not ..push your way through to the front ranks of your profession; do not run after.. rewards.. find an entry into the world of beauty."
> Konstantin Stanislavsky

10 YEAR 2000: DISAGREEMENT OVER TRAINING CHANGES

Content
Reaction to New Staff
Leadership Models
NHS Reform – Satellite Teams run by Clinicians
Finding Identity in Large Organisations
Masters Degree in Mental Health
Terminology - Trades and Professions
Historical Aspects of NHS Unqualified Workers
Knowledge and Skills Framework
The National Occupational Standards (NOS)
Graduate Mental Health Worker
Clinical Nurse Specialist

Reaction to New Staff

Medicine is the oldest profession and over time has become a powerful institution. Many staff are long-standing and therefore gained a great deal of power by dint of knowledge of systems and networks. When a new discipline appears such institutionalized staff react in many ways:

- fear having their authority challenged
- welcome the challenge of new ideas
- be suspicious of newcomers
- welcome a load-sharing facility
- be concerned about new treatments
- try to gain ownership of favourite or influential patients / clients
- become gatekeepers to keep newcomers out
- develop anxiety about newcomers qualifications
- welcome or discredit newcomers

How staff react to newcomers depends to a great degree on the type of leadership they have. During my time in three mental health teams, only one had a strong Manager but even there staff were pressured to 'follow' group thinking. We should never underestimate the power of groups, the very different behaviours evinced to the usual modus operandi of individuals comprising it. I have witnessed and been the target of bullying among such teams and it is soul destroying. That is why it is vital to gain an understanding of how such things happen and prevent scapegoating.

Leadership Models

A person who facilitates a group and enables its growth is more often referred to as a leader than a manager. Leadership, in my view, is vital within an NHS which can become a grinding machine with burned out employees and blaming instead of co-operation. The movie 'Metropolis' and book '1984' depict the suffering in bad organizations. It is a constant struggle to deal with 21st century life and work is a large part of that stress.

The new cohorts (body of students) of Degree-taking Mental Health Workers might find themselves in this position if they do not have adequate and well-trained team leaders. It is the Team Leader's job to explain the dynamics of groups to staff and be active in the reconciliation of new and old ideas. Leadership is little understood but vital for building decent workplaces. Well lead, organized teams welcome rather than stigmatize and prevent scapegoating or bullying.

I heard it said by a man training a group of horticulturists with learning difficulties that although his trainees were ready for the community, the community was not ready for them. I believe this is true of people with severe mental health problems. Teams of colleagues like social communities will only 'become ready' when individual members are fulfilled and work together to deal with the few who cause aggravation, most often to talented newcomers. If you have any doubt this happens, see my anti bullying blog. 14000 NHS staff have been bullied out of post, according to research, from their toxic workplaces.

There is a growing call for organisations without traditional managers, which are run on a co-operative basis by staff working on an equal basis. Such a model would work well in organizations such as the UK NHS.

NHS Reform – Satellite Teams run by Clinicians

Clinician-lead small teams is an NHS model put forward by respected American Doctor, Dr Susan Parenti. Her paper appears at the back of this book. Dr Parenti believes in small is beautiful, a growing movement in the UK. Dr Parenti believes change is possible from clinicians on the inside. She moots the idea of perturbation – ripples and slight movements which cause changes for the better, without ill feeling or violent opposition. David CAN win Goliath; by strategy, fairness and determination. I urge you to read this paper, sharing it with colleagues and friends.

Figure 12 Psychology of Change

Prochaska and DiClemente's trans-theoretical model of behaviour change. This model shows an individual's journey towards accepting change. It demonstrates the ambivalence and learning cycles, which can hamper as

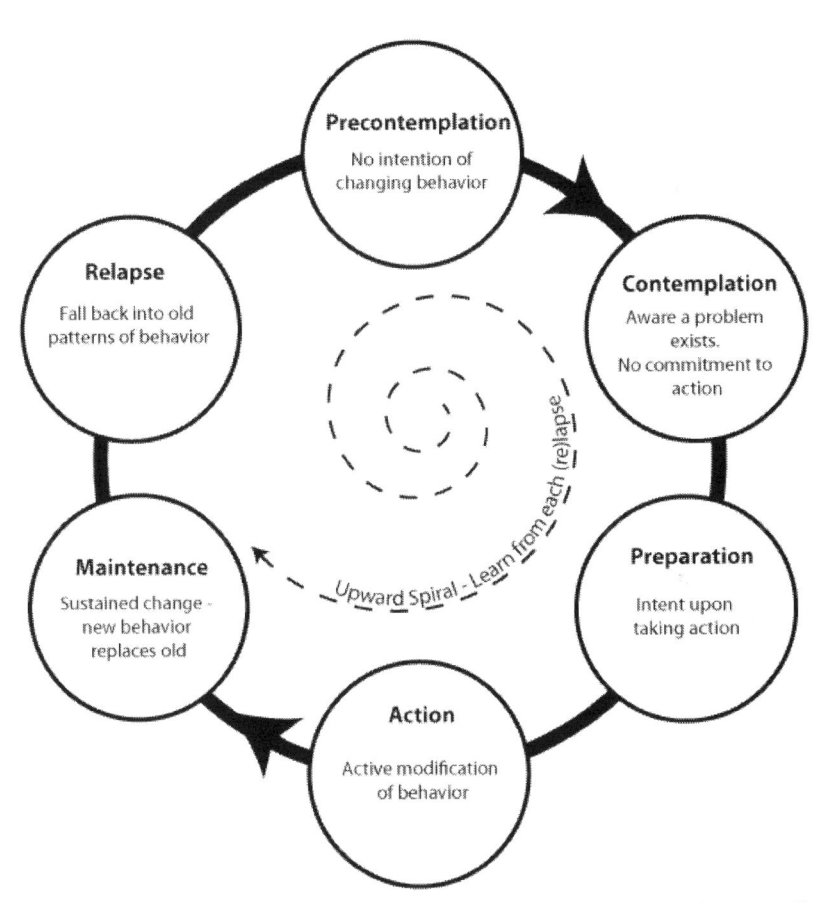

```
         Precontemplation
         No intention of
         changing behavior

Relapse                        Contemplation
Fall back into old             Aware a problem
patterns of behavior           exists.
                               No commitment to
                               action

         Upward Spiral - Learn from each (re)lapse

Maintenance                    Preparation
Sustained change -             Intent upon
new behavior                   taking action
replaces old

              Action
         Active modification
            of behavior
```

well as take success forward. In group settings, each individual is struggling with this same model, which makes the success of implementation of change more difficult, unless strongly managed by good leadership skills. The model demonstrates the cyclic nature of change and how learning can be made from relapses. But the model also works in reverse mode. This is where groups diversify, argue and find scapegoats and become toxic.

Finding Identity in Large Organisations

Trying to maintain identity, especially if you are far from family or social support is not easy even in this age of easy communication. Building better communities needs people who care about the environment and ALL the people who live there; whatever their perceived ability, disability or differences.

Your identity in the NHS was once merely a matter of which profession you had chosen. This is no longer so. With roles blurring and reforming over time (I call this the kaleidoscope effect) something more was necessary. Individuals were expected to work in Dickensian clinical settings and dealing, without adequate support, traumatized families, newly diagnosed patients, complex problems and abuse. Mental health workers cannot do these things without a strong sense of who you are, where you belong in the system and access to good support networks.

I have been traumatized by my experiences at the hands of rogue Managers and staff, but hope I am not bitter. I make no bones about how difficult it was to survive ten years ago, in teams of traditionalists who opposed change and being lone representative of a new guard. As I went through this three times before leaving the NHS for good, I count myself an expert by experience. Only much passing time and reflection has allowed me to review my experiences at a distance. The NHS never catered for individuals who questioned methods, for whatever reason. The NHS was and is a microcosm of the community and subject to the same petty boilings-up over nothing; not surprising given its twin towers of poor finance and professional rivalry. Typically, whenever change was introduced into the NHS, it happened quickly, and without proper advice and training, leaving staff to flounder. Education as always was the missing link.

Introduce new ideas into a group and put an individual into that group who represents this change, what do you expect will happen? It is not the individual who is targeted per se, but what they represent. Anyone who says otherwise, ask them how stigma comes about –the same factors are at play, the unknown, the feared, the imagined. This is not just the NHS as the model can be fitted to any institution or organization which has been in existence many years with few major changes in management. The problem itself points to the answer.

Masters Degree in Mental Health

Several cohorts of students had taken the Masters in Mental Health by the time I walked out of the NHS. It was offered on 3 levels; 1st year Certificate and practice, 3rd year Diploma, 4th year Masters. Unfortunately funding was cut so the promised PhD's were not forthcoming.

figure 13 Tuckman Model: Group Behaviour During Changes

This model shows groups during the process of change. This applies to new groups and those encountering major change. In all cases, the storming or arguing stage is inevitable. This is where, without leadership, scapegoating of change agent(s) or representative(s) of the new idea(s) is inevitable.

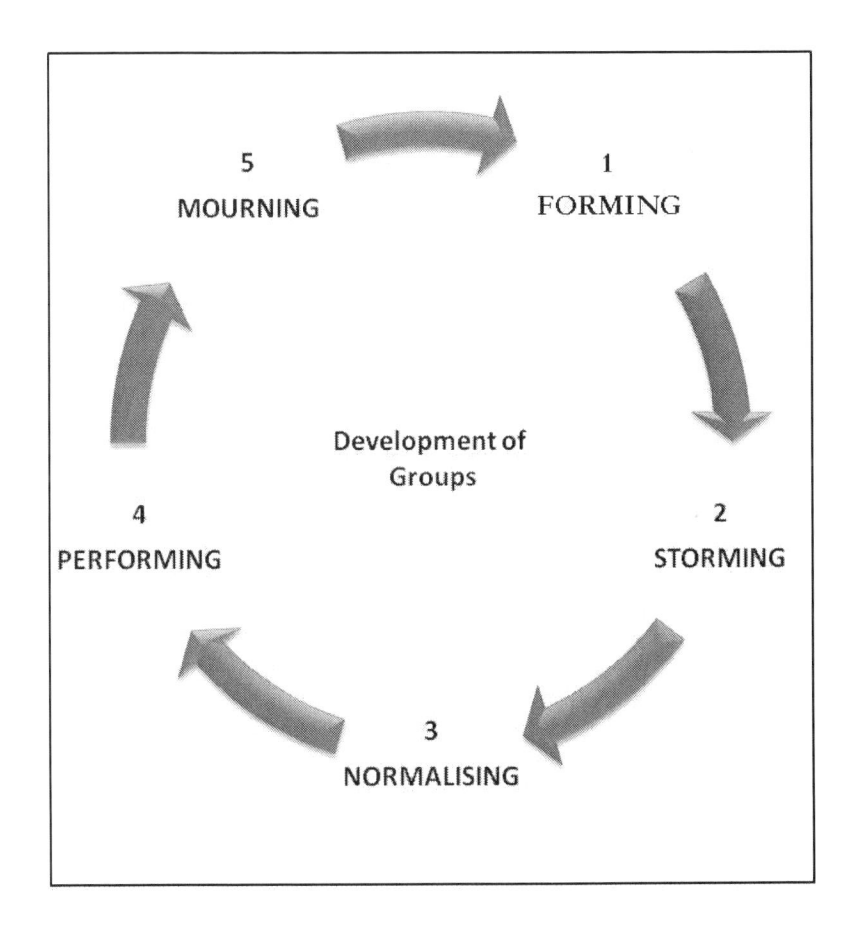

Development of Groups

1. FORMING
2. STORMING
3. NORMALISING
4. PERFORMING
5. MOURNING

The Government intended the Degree as starting point for all mental health professionals; Doctor to Health Care Assistant. Professional qualifications were to be branches off the degree. The skills and knowledge which this course covered were:
- Government mental health policy
- NHS implementation of policy
- mental health and the law
- links between statutory and voluntary organisations
- fundamentals of mental illness
- theoretical stances and the role of professionals
- theory of different types of therapy and practice
- the process of research

Naturally, this was a controversial development, especially among long-term staff who were anxious about their future careers. It was intended that traditional roles (psychiatry, nursing) would exist side by side with new roles, some which would be created as local need demanded. This would have created a service that was both national and local in structure at the same time. It would have been a huge undertaking and was just getting off the ground after fine efforts by University trainers. Whatever the roles become, they will be pioneering. Pioneering calls for sacrifice and the need to work together; a task that calls for mature personalities with enthusiasm and confidence. I will say no more.

Terminology - Trades and Professions

Before I begin talking about the basis of the career routes planned I want to consider the snobbishness that comes with the use of the terms trade and profession. Ah, one must also count among the professions the humble prostitute, the oldest profession apart from the law..

Being of working class stock, I was brought up alongside tradesmen of all kinds, so I am in a good position to present a rounded view, especially since my education puts me in the middle classes. I use the term trade because I would like to de-stigmatize it. Trades are what artisans do to earn a living; carpenter, bricklayer, boat builder, miner, electrician. These are skilled trades requiring much knowledge, experience and having their own peculiar language and tools. The term trade has been stigmatized for a very long time.

In the 17th century all non-conformists were barred from University. Members of the Society of Friends (Quakers; followers of George Fox) were de-barred from entering the traditional professions of law, teaching and the church. Instead they turned their hand to trade. Quakers became very successful at trade and as a result grew rich.

Figure 14 Lewin's Unified Field Theory (1920's)

This diagram shows inter-group arguments, the dynamics of change between old and new, and how scapegoats / rival groups are attacked by authoritarian groups with mediator groups attempting to integrate ideas.

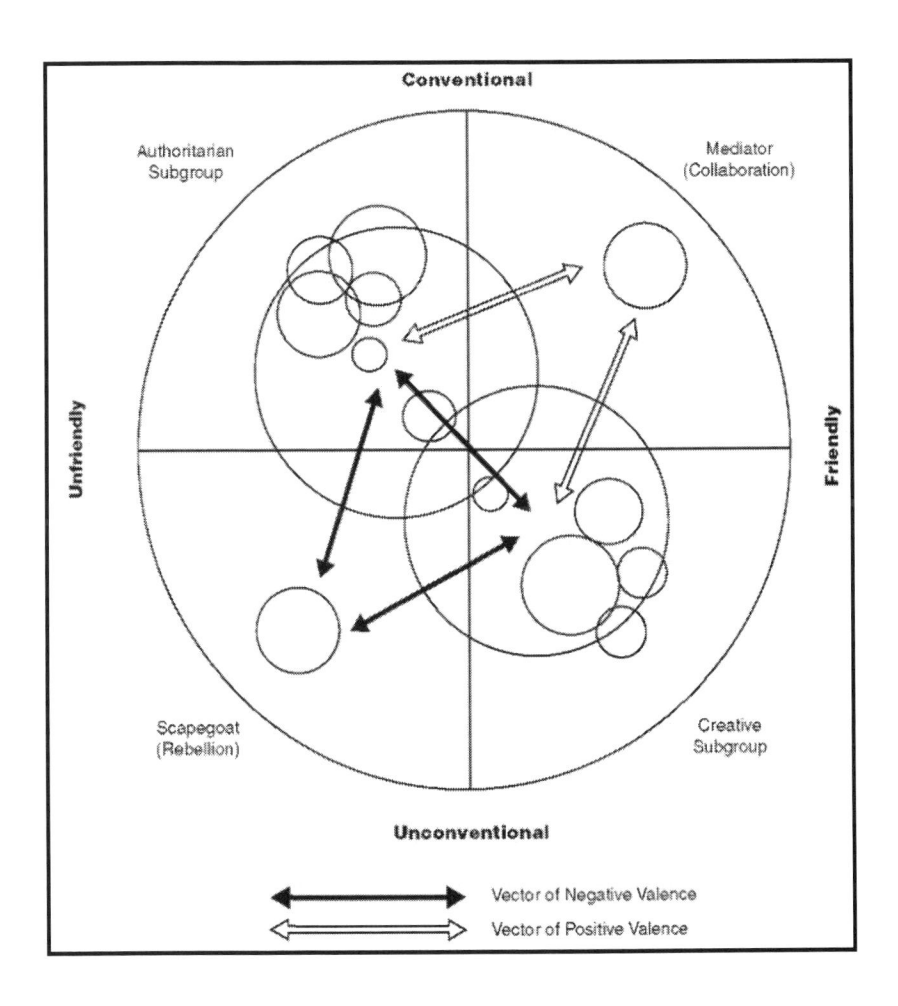

Most of you know the names Fry, Cadbury and Barclay. These families were not only rich and successful but became great philanthropists, because they did not separate their religious from their temporal lives.

Trade is still somewhat looked down upon, as if it is less valuable than profession. The truth is, were it not for skilled trades, society would not exist. Without engineers and plumbers we would long ago have succumbed to disease. So, for the duration of this book, please understand if I prefer the term trade to profession.

Historical Aspects of NHS Unqualified Workers

If you joined the NHS at its beginnings you had a choice of two trades: Doctor or Nurse. Later, Psychologist, Social Worker and Occupational Therapist were added. If you could afford training, the world was your oyster. If you could not, you might be able to find a job and train in what amounted to an apprenticeship; working on-the-job for a pittance and receive training at the same time. If you had no money and could persuade someone to take you as a vocational trainee, you might be given an assistant role in Social Work, Occupational Therapy, Healthcare or perhaps an Auxiliary Nursing post. If you were unlucky (and many were) you would remain in your lowly role for years and, despite hard-won knowledge and skills, remain on unqualified pay scales. I was 7 years in this position, followed by another 2 years as a Counsellor on half wages. By the time I left St John's Hospital, Rehabilitation Officers had been given the opportunity to take NVQ in Care, which took them on to qualified pay scales. There are far more opportunities, in theory, providing budgets do not run out.

Knowledge and Skills Framework

If you look at the descriptions of trades in previous chapters you will notice how many overlap. This is partly why staff were fearful of change - in case they lost status. There are many areas of knowledge and skill in each of the mental health trades. The Government realized this and started to look at different elements of the work and break them into components. They came up with something City & Guilds students would recognise; a framework of knowledge and skills, broken into elements each with a definition and means of proving they had successfully completed each task.
Communication
- Personal and people development
- Health, safety and security
- Service improvement
- Quality
- Equality and diversity

Such a system would have made it possible for anyone to learn the elements of the framework and gain a qualification. Ah, you may say, I can understand communication is vital in mental health, also health and safety; but how does that qualify someone to become a mental health worker? Well it does because that is only part of the equation.

The National Occupational Standards (NOS)

Working in parallel with the Knowledge and Skills Framework were the National Occupational Standards (NOS) which define all key areas of mental health work. For example, to work with mental health patients you have to be able to reflect on your own behaviour. So, there are standards which define what reflection means. Once a candidate has proved they can reflect, that forms part of the qualification. It might be easier if we looked at one example.

Standard - practice in reflective & professionally appropriate manner
1. relating to and interacting with individuals
2. identifying the relationship needs of individuals
3. developing effective relationship with a patient
4. monitoring and altering the relationships to meet changing needs

So, you might ask, how do I prove I've done these? There are many ways. For example, in 3. 'developing effective relationship with a patient' - you might:

- write an essay about your experiences with a patient
- ask your supervisor to provide a testimonial
- produce a patient testimonial or letter of thanks
- ask a colleague to write a testimonial of your patient work

Ah, you might say, but anyone can write anything; how do the examiners know it's true? Tutors are wise and come to know your strengths and weaknesses. You are not expected to be perfect, only capable of learning - you are allowed mistakes! You need to bring to class situations that have not worked well and demonstrate how you learned from those and what you would do differently. Anyone who cannot brook positive criticism and consider alternative ways of resolving problems has a REAL problem and should not be working in mental health.

Passing K&S and NOS are not like passing exams by swotting from a book but hands-on elements of everyday work. The NOS are the highway code of mental health. They are skills to be proud of. There are many ways of gaining the information to do this work:

- Certificate, Diploma & Masters in Mental Health
- professional development through add-on training and certificates
- specialist training e.g. qualifying to prescribe requires specialist study

- a surgeon practices on cadavers (dead bodies)
- talking-cure therapists are given ongoing supervision
- trainees can practice on colleagues [this can be fun]

Phew, that's enough about training. Let's look at what working in these trades involves. As all was new in 2000 when the Degree was frozen, there were not many advertised posts. I shall give two examples of the posts that were on offer at this time.

Graduate Mental Health Worker

There were no formal qualifications for entry but interviews and written tests for potential Graduate Mental Health Workers. Candidates with a mental health background or qualification were preferred but it was not prerequisite. A mature attitude and broad life experience was vital. This new post was set up nation-wide as a result of specific Government funding. Mental health workers were to work in hospitals, community or Primary Care. Some would have gone on to train as clinicians others to work in community projects; anything from helping set up a green gym, logging services in the area or working with mental health patients.

Clinical Nurse Specialist

Clinical Nurse Specialists were consultant grade nurses working in the field for years with extensive knowledge of their trade. They worked as nurses and specialist consultants, some starting local service initiatives, for example children and family working. Some of these nurses took additional training so they could prescribe, others intended to specialize in research.

****

So, that was the situation during the Government initiative of 2000, which began to go wrong and then had funding cuts. Gradually and slowly the situation improved and Mental Health Workers and the new brief therapy system in Primary Care is beginning to roll out, albeit there is still much opposition.

At this point, you might read Dr Parenti's paper at Appendix 1. This was her suggestion for reform of the US healthcare system, giving better access by poor patients and changing top heavy management to small teams of clinicians with their own budgets. Read it and consider if it would work in the UK NHS.

> 'Even the smallest person can change the course of the future.'
> Lord of the Rings. J R R Tolkien

11   AFTERCARE

Content
Aftercare
Dealing with Facts: There is No Cure
Support for Enduring Mental Illness
Assertive Outreach
Rehabilitation Units
Support for Day Patients
Self Help
Counselling Charitable Organisations
Therapeutic Communities

Aftercare
Once diagnosis has been achieved and a care plan put into action, professionals follow up with continuing aftercare, in order to prevent relapse. Unfortunately this vital stage has often been missed leading to unfortunate events which triggered negative press about mentally ill patients. At this moment in time, it is impossible to predict the likelihood of relapse. Until this becomes possible, aftercare remains a vital part of the treatment plan.

Dealing with Facts: There is No Cure
There is no cure for mental illness because there is no cure for life. We must all regard ourselves as being in remission, whether from schizophrenia or stress. There are several positive things about this way of thinking:
1. awareness of a condition leads to better self care
2. monitoring your own mental health is a preventative
3. the more we learn, the more we maintain control of a situation

There is a certain equality in realizing everyone will have to deal with stress' whether or not that leads onto to further mental illness. Everyone will deal with bereavement or loss, known factors in depression. No one is the perfect human. Somewhere in your patient's system, in fact all of our systems, is an Achilles heel, whether that is physical, spiritual or mental.

The prevalence of depression is 1:4 and that of schizophrenia 1:25. There are many people with undiagnosed personality disorders. People who believe themselves perfect are most likely to have a problem whereas awareness, without fear, of mental problems is most likely to bring help. The word normal is a measure but has no other meaning. We have already looked at the danger of assuming someone else is 'ill' and that we are not.

Support for Enduring Mental Illness

There is very little in the way of aftercare, except for known patients with long standing mental illness. For such patients there are excellent services provided by mental health charities, providing many volunteers and care workers who tirelessly work on behalf of their clientele. In the NHS, our crumbling bastion of an antiquated system, there are Community Mental Health Teams, comprising a mixed range of professionals:

- Psychiatrists
- Mental nurses
- Psychologists
- Social workers
- Occupational Therapists

Currently they treat patients and referrals from Primary Care. I described these teams more fully in Understanding Mental Illness. Rivalries were always rife in these teams. Hopefully, when the new mental health worker grades start filtering through the system, so that everyone has equal training at the start of their career, the outworn sense of superiority will melt away. I hope so.

Assertive Outreach and teams set up to deal with early intervention methods for psychosis also offer support to chronically ill patients who are known to have regular relapse patterns. Within communities, there are **Rehabilitation Units**, for patients who need some support but can live for a short time before being re-settled within the community. The last of the patients from asylum days are now long dead. These pioneers of community living undertook all the anxieties and difficulties that entailed. They were the end of an era for the treatment of mental illness. We should not forget them.

Support for Day Patients

In the last few years Primary Care GP's had taken on Counsellors in their surgeries but these have, over time, been replaced by the stepped care programme, which offers interventions ranging from stress management courses to through group therapy to individuals sessions, depending upon the severity of the problems on a need basis.

At your GP surgery, you might ask to be referred for counselling but be offered no more than four to six sessions on the brief therapy model so once derided (forgive me my need to gloat, but I underwent a considerable amount of suffering as a pioneer in this model). There is no choice over therapist in Primary Care.

Figure 15 We Must Never Forget Asylum Patients

Asylum patients must never be forgotten. They were real people, pioneers for the field where you are working or volunteering or being treated with proper respect as a patient. These people underwent much suffering, ridicule, loneliness, ignored by families, forgotten by the community and used as experimental guinea pigs by early Physicians.
Please keep them in your remembrance.

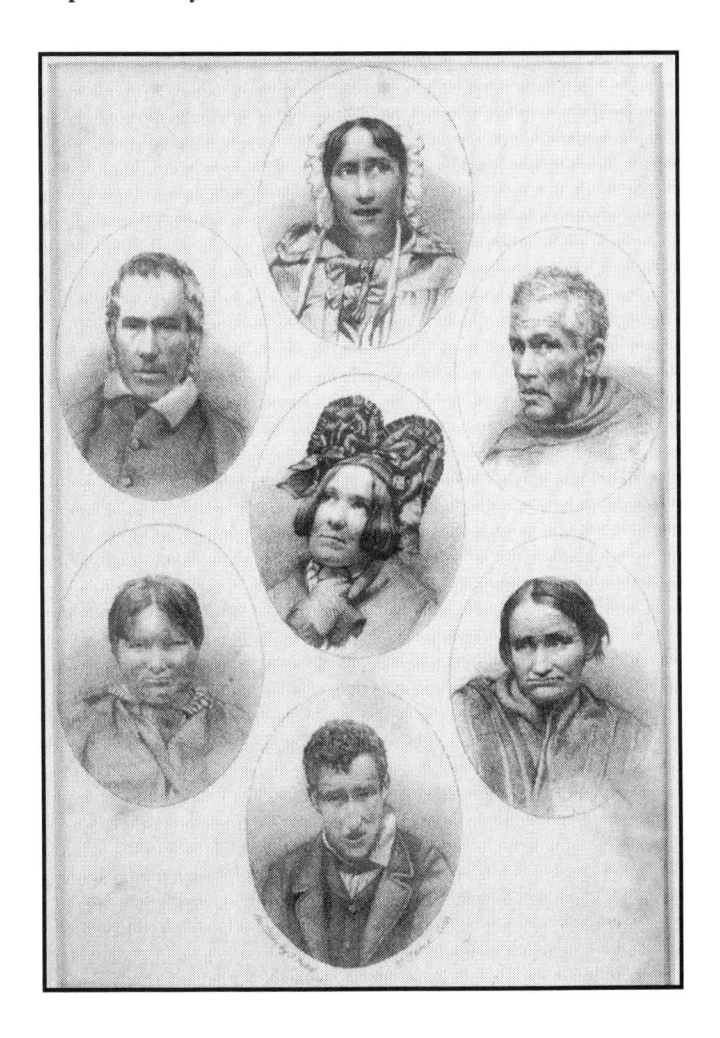

Although brief therapy is useful for short term or emotional problems, it does not resolve problems which need in-depth supportive counselling or psychotherapy; for example abuse, bullying, severe emotional problems, bereavement, autism support (i.e. for the stress which attends autism) or chronic depressive illness.

Self Help

There is one avenue of support which has been growing and that is information easily available to download from the Internet. Our American cousins are very organised in that respect and you can find a great deal of useful information free of charge. However, do watch what you recommend to patients. Stick to mental health charities and universities, pukka news sites like the BBC or professional ones like the Royal College of Psychiatrists who provide free information leaflets for home printing.

Counselling Charitable Organisations

Many counselling charitable organisations started off with good intention, to provide trainees with training which was paid for by charitable donations (trainees were still expected to provide a donation and to give free services on completion of training for a fixed period). Their trainees now charge NHS patients at private fee rates, using NHS rooms in Primary Care often for free. They say these rates pay for the service but they also cover the cost of administration, offices etc. Their reduced rates are steep, considering impoverished people are on national minimum wage or benefits, but there are few avenues these days for free counselling, which is a great shame. Sometimes brief therapy does not plug the gap, and in chronic life problems just does not work, I'm afraid, as this requires longer term input.

Therapeutic Communities

As a sort of response to public anxiety about personality disordered mentally ill patients. I want to briefly cover therapeutic communities.

Therapeutic communities cater for those who do not have the social skills to live in the community, but can be helped to enjoy more organised, productive lives and better relationships. They are mainly personality disordered patients, frequently imprisoned and often from abusive families. I mentioned one well known therapeutic community in HMP Grendon, which won an award for their work in this area. There is not much research in the effectiveness of this treatment but that which has been carried out gives positive results. Patients and staff live together on an equal basis, with decisions shared by both.

Figure 16 Therapeutic Communities

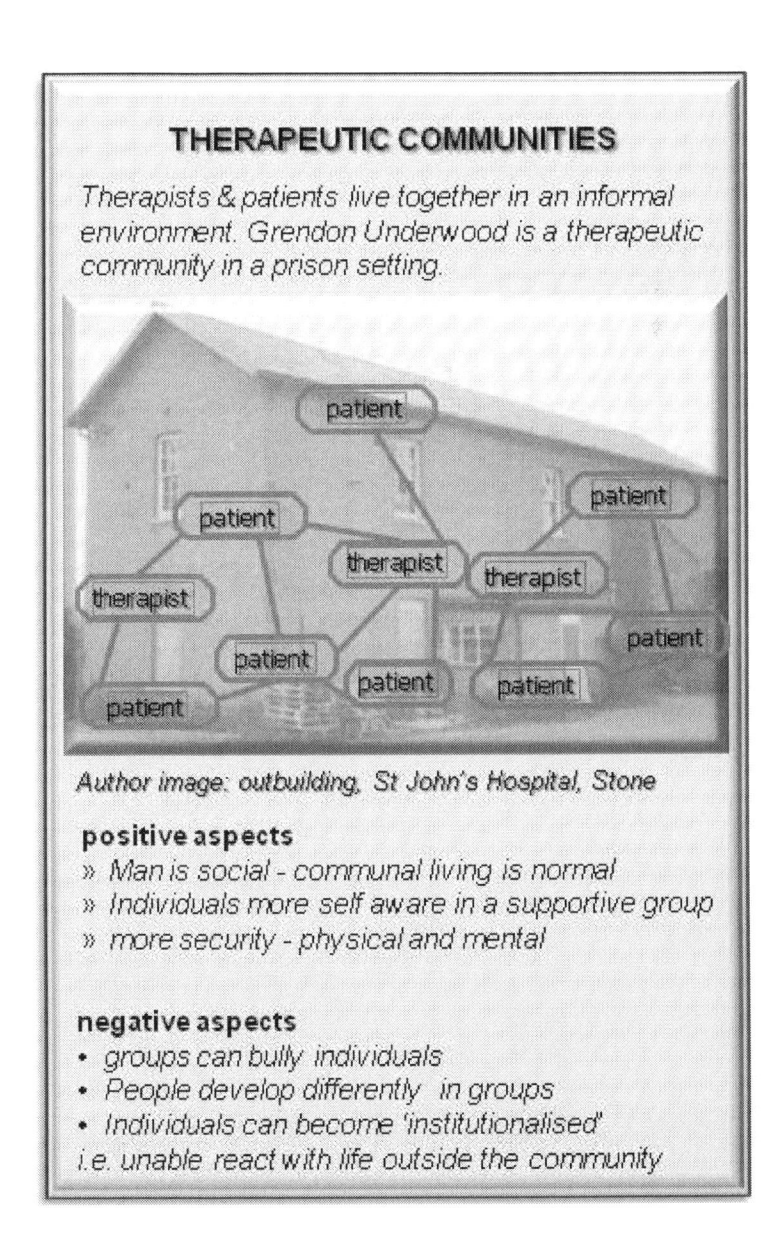

THERAPEUTIC COMMUNITIES

Therapists & patients live together in an informal environment. Grendon Underwood is a therapeutic community in a prison setting.

Author image: outbuilding, St John's Hospital, Stone

positive aspects
» Man is social - communal living is normal
» Individuals more self aware in a supportive group
» more security - physical and mental

negative aspects
• groups can bully individuals
• People develop differently in groups
• Individuals can become 'institutionalised'
i.e. unable react with life outside the community

A great deal of self-disclosure is required and all patients are expected to join therapy groups, individual analysis, work and social events. Emphasis is on learning social skills and having unacceptable behaviours brought in the open so patients become aware of maladaptive behaviours. The community can reject those who refuse to obey the rules. This seems, in principle, to answer the needs of this group for a place in a society, modification of behaviour and a sense of belonging which this group of patients are unlikely to have experienced.

There are always outcries or moral panics against prisoner-patients but little sense of understanding of why they are as they are. These people, usually male, are the outcasts of society. I am not asking they be loved and liked, because most people find this impossible, just that humanity can be extended to a group who had their lives taken away at an early age and have probably experienced little happiness or companionship. As a caring society, can we exclude anyone, whatever they are deemed to have done?

There are positive and negative factors at play in living in a therapeutic community.

Positive
- man is a social being - living in communities is the norm.
- individuals are more self-aware in a supportive group, with mental and physical security

Negative
- groups can scapegoat individuals
- people develop different characteristics in groups to when they live alone
- patients and therapists can become institutionalised

****

Key Learning
- No Cure - there is no cure for mental illness. Awareness is likely to reduce symptoms as is stability and social support.
- NHS Aftercare - resources lacking but often given by volunteers
- Brief Therapy - popular in NHS but not a panacea for long-term issues.
- Self Help - popular, often free by way of books, Internet and libraries.
- Therapeutic Communities – provide care for marginalised patients; for example, patients and prisoners with severe personality disorder.

> 'helping academics find .. that different publics have sophisticated, interesting ideas that can challenge them, surprise them, help them think: that's a profound message.
> Professor Kathy Sykes, Science Communication

12   EVIDENCE V EXPERIENCE

Content
Quality Control in Therapies
About Medical, Complementary & Alternatives
Lack of Funding
National Institute for Health & Clinical Excellence [NICE]
Social Care Centre for Excellence [SCIE]
Evidence Base in Primary Care
The Need for Research
Therapeutic Relationship and Placebo
Medication in Mental Health

In this chapter, I briefly cover the regulatory machinery of medical and therapeutic treatments which ensure that:
➢ patients are not cheated
➢ standards are maintained
➢ new treatments are tested and approved
➢ no patient is harmed by treatments
➢ therapists practice in an ethical manner

I call the chapter 'experiment v experience' because there are two ways we can find out if things work (are effective):
➢ experiment – research
➢ experience –doing or receiving the treatment

Western medicine is generally based on experiment whilst Eastern medicine values experience. None of these are the right way; it depends what is being tested. If potentially dangerous chemicals are being concocted in a laboratory for consumption by the public, there needs to be legislation for its manufacture and a license for its sale. Research is carried out on chemicals, practitioners prescribing must be regulated, drugs need to be licensed to show they are safe.

If patients are offered therapeutic services like healing or counselling there need to be ethical guidelines to ensure patients are treated with respect. Therapeutic practice must be underpinned with training. It is true that, pre-umbrella days, practitioners were practicing on the basis of extensive patient experience. Their effectiveness was proven by the fact they remained in business! This is still the case in many alternative treatments. The field of talking cures is relatively new and still being regulated. But hopefully it will not become over-regulated as some organisations are, which cuts out innovation. On the other hand, training is no assurance of effectiveness, ethics or quality. I have experienced both sides of the coin; individuals clearly well qualified but lacked basic life nous and so-called unqualified Therapists who did more for me than many a GP.

Quality Control in Therapies

In all purchased services we have forms of quality control to make sure customers are not cheated and goods are kept up to standard. In ancient medical history, quality control comprised the priest Ugg being clubbed to death or Inzar the priestess buried alive by angry mobs if rituals were not effective. Nowadays statutory and voluntary bodies act on punters' behalf in marginally less vindictive ways for example:

- Government public health regulations
- National Institute for Health & Clinical Effectiveness (NICE)
- Social Care Institute for Excellence (SCIE)
- legislative instruments (policy)
- British Medical Association (BMA)
- Mind, the mental health charity
- Carers UK

Those with large means have access to Courts and as a last resort to local and national media, as well as professional umbrella associations. By the latter I do not mean purveyors of rain protective equipment but organisations which represent the schools within the professions. Each profession has its own umbrella (e.g. British Association for Counselling, which covers counselling and Psychotherapy). Unfortunately there are so many such bodies it is virtually impossible to know all of them. What happens mostly is you learn of the ones you need and others filter in through media, contacts and research.

Lack of Funding

The Government has little funding for research projects although their ideal is complete regulation (hence, control over) all treatments. Over-regulation is not always for the right reasons, i.e. best care of patients. Traditional medicine and therapies have regulatory bodies, training and umbrella organisations. These often have large numbers of staff in well appointed buildings and charge phenomenal membership fees.

This system excludes good therapists. They either have to give up their career or work at several other jobs at the same time as practicing therapy. Although we do not like to acknowledge the class system I'm afraid it still exists – it is a therapeutic class ceiling and caused by lack of income not pre-ordained status.

As more and more therapies are regulated, this squeezes out smaller but excellent training schools who cannot afford the fees demanded by umbrella organisations.

The Government long ago began talks with BAC to try to make counselling less elitist by reducing onerous training requirements for accreditation. The cost of supervision, rooms and insurance is so onerous that counsellors have to charge high fees to stay in business. Even NHS Primary Care is getting in on the act, with high room hire rates charged by cash strapped Practice Managers who are adding to the problematic situation. Unfortunately, this situation at the end of the day means that patients who need counselling are unable to find affordable treatment.

National Institute for Health & Clinical Excellence (NICE)

NICE is an organization set up as a result of the 2004 white paper, Choosing Health: Making Health Choices Easier. The Government wanted to bring together knowledge and guidance on promoting good health, as well as treating ill health. Like the Government, NICE uses independent advisory groups comprised of professionals and lay people who have an interest in or experience of mental health issues.

NICE offers guidance on clinical practice, the use of new and existing medicines and treatments in the NHS. The Department of Health refer specific health issues to NICE, who look at the evidence and develop recommendations for (for example) the use of medications or preparations intended for patient prescriptions in Primary Care. Clinical guidelines are a form of standard which ensure that effective treatments are offered patients. For example, Cognitive Behavioral Therapy and Brief Therapy (solution focused) have been ratified by NICE as treatments of choice in Primary Care for patients with depressive illness.

NICE, like all NHS organizations, has limited funds and so resources are scarce. Funds are spent on developing guidelines on conditions that affect large groups of people, such as depression and anxiety or which have a significant impact on the health of the population, such as obesity. For social care, there is an equivalent organization called the Social Care Institute for Excellence (SCIE).

Social Care Centre for Excellence (SCIE)

Unlike NICE, SCIE enjoys charitable status and is independent of the Government, although it was set up by them in 2001, to improve how social care is delivered, by offering good practice guidance. SCIE is supported by the Department of Health as well as the Department for Education and Skills (DfES) and is run by a Board of Trustees. There are two main organisational arms:

- The Partners' Council - comprises 40 organisations connected with health issues e.g. patient, carer, research institutes, who advise SCIE on priority issues
- The Practice Partners' Network - has a circle of member organisations from statutory, voluntary and private sectors, who share experiences on good practice.

So, what other factors do we need to consider around the area of treatments before we dive into the nitty-gritty of details? One is the surprising but often forgotten facts around basic premises which are used (sometimes exploited by) practitioners. These three have long been known to medics.

- therapeutic relationship
- placebo effect
- hope

Therapeutic Relationship and Placebo

The therapeutic relationship should not be undervalued. It is recognised as a vital process in therapy as is the patient's belief system. In Understanding Mental Illness I described how there is a blind trial in drug trials, where some participants are given an inert substance instead of the drug being tested. This ensures that benefits of the drug cannot be ascribed to patient belief (what is called placebo effect).

The link between patient belief and cure is fascinating and needs research. It is accepted by physicians that positive therapeutic relationship and placebo effect both have a bearing on successful outcome. Another word you might use for placebo is hope. A Channel 4 programme by Professor Kathy Sykes explored this in depth. During laying-on-of-hands healing sessions, CAT scans showed patients pain centres visibly diminishing. This demonstrates the physical benefit of therapeutic relationships between healer and patient, whether you believe it is the relationship itself or some as yet unknown healing force of the healer.

Medication in Mental Health

I explored the process of drug trials in Understanding Mental Illness. It takes up to a decade for a new drug to progress from first discovery to being made available to the public. This may shorten as virtual trials [computer simulation] start to become feasible. Psychiatric drugs were a relatively new innovation in the 1950's. Some of the earliest were:

- Largactil in syrup form - reduces psychotic symptoms
- Anti depressants – raises mood in depressive illness
- Lithium - levels mood in mania
- Haloperidol – used in the treatment of psychosis

Figure 17 SCIE Services

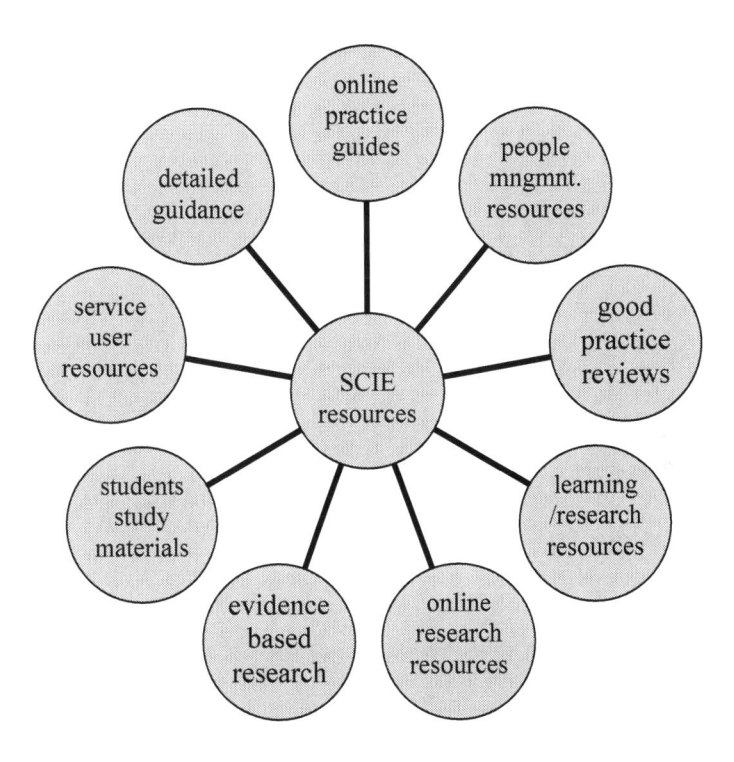

The discovery of anti-depressants is a good example of serendipity (where a discovery is made through accident). Nurses on tuberculosis wards noticed how certain drugs were making patients jubilant. Around the same time, work was being done by scientists on chemical transmitters in the brain, and how these affected mood levels. Some insightful scientists started to put these facts together and eventually drugs being used for tuberculosis were synthesised into anti-depressants.

By the 1960's, the tranquillisers Librium and Valium were commonly prescribed, particularly to women, for nervous disorders. These were withdrawn from use when they were found to be addictive.

Anti-depressant medication is commonly used for anxiety disorders. Prozac became popular in the treatment of depression. Later, the SSRI class drugs fell from grace when drugs regulatory authorities discovered that a side effect was increasing suicidal ideation (though pharmaceutical giants Lilley, who produced Prozac, denied this).

Many people do not like synthesised (laboratory made) medication and prefer natural remedies, despite the fact that there is only anecdotal evidence for their effectiveness. St John's Wort is one of the better known remedies used for relieving symptoms of depression and is commonly available in pharmacies.

****

Key Learning
- evidence v experience - two ways of learning; evidence (research, science) and experience (working with patients).
- changing styles of treatment - NHS now accepting complementary treatments as patients exercise choice away from trad medicine.
- class ceiling in therapy – this is down to the extortionate cost of training, professional development and supervision.
- why no affordable therapy - training and cost at the heart of a lack of affordable therapy for patients.
- evidence based care - NHS bodies responsible for evidence bases for care are NICE and SCIE.
- therapeutic relationship, placebo, hope - topics related to empathy and belief; both powerful healing qualities.
- medication in mental illness - widely used to alleviate symptoms in psychosis, mania, depression, which do not readily respond to talking cures.

> 'It is better to learn wisdom late, than not at all'
> Conan Doyle, The Man with the Twisted Lip

13 GRADUATE MENTAL HEALTH WORKERS

Content
What do Graduate mental health workers do?
Informal Rules For Mental Health Workers

What do Graduate mental health workers do?

I remember asking this rhetorical question years ago, when I entered the field. I guess the answer has not changed. Although formal direction and qualifications were lacking, the truth upon which we based our work was to enable anyone with active mental illness to live fulfilled lives in the community. I remember feeling lost until I started reading and studying for myself. It was one thing helping someone fill in housing or benefit forms, listening to relationship problems or existential life problems, quite another to help a stranger find their way towards fulfilment. You can go on courses, listen to colleagues and supervisors, read extensively, but it will only start to make sense when you have overcome some major problem in your own life. So, although I can't describe what you are meant to do in your work, I offer you my own rules.

Informal Rules For Mental Health Workers

1. Reflection and Personal Experience - One cannot divorce life experience from practice. To do so would be folly. It is the ability to reflect and distance oneself that makes the difference.
2. Listen to the Patient - Do not bandy clinical terms or label people. How would you feel if someone called you a depressive? Try to understand your patient's situation; environment, culture and personal beliefs. Don't label someone because they behave differently to your expectations.
3. Don't Put Up with Jargon - Jargon has its place, in being a kind of shorthand. However, it can be used to baffle or control rather than aid understanding. Some people use jargon because they think it sounds grand. It doesn't. Anyone who can't explain in simple terms does not understand the subject themselves.
4. Equality - There needs to be an equal relationship between therapist and patient. There is something wrong with a professional who demands a power differential.
5. Be Cautious of Taking Credit - If you take credit for what goes right, you need to accept blame for what goes wrong. The better path is to guide; offer the patient a map and a compass. This is all you can do.

6. Safeguard Your Heart - Do not offer patients your heart nor over-concern for their welfare. Protect yourself with a barrier lest their pain breach your heart.
7. Patients Are Human, Not Always Kind - Patients are not always kind people. They are human and will fail as you fail. They will antagonise or speak negatively about you. They are not always honest or nice. You need to understand why.
8. Finding Professional Support - Find support where you can; trustworthy peers, good training and most of all an experienced supervisor not afraid to tell the truth. These will be rare people.
9. There Are Many Injustices - Do not believe all is sweetness and light in this field for it is not. It reflects life and life has its injustices. Do not become despondent, because the work is its own reward. Often, it may be the only reward.
10. Patient Sensitivity and Dignity - Patients have human rights; they do not have to give information or fill in forms. Do not force them to do so.
11. Eliciting Information Can Be Difficult - Getting information out of someone who does not know you and is afraid of symptoms (and of you) is not easy. Find a balance between getting information without leaving the patient embarrassed or diminished. Remember:

➢ patients give information in different ways
➢ diagnoses or assessments can take more than one visit
➢ information is not given in a linear way

i.e. you may have a list of questions but the patient will not offer their story in that order. Do not make them repeat because you failed to take adequate notes.

It is easy for mental health workers to forget the patient is firstly a fellow human being with a life outside their illness. I can't count the number of times I have heard so-called professionals saying things like;

☹ 'I'll slot you in this appointment..'
☹ 'I'll see you on Friday at 2pm..' (no choice offered)]
☹ 'she's a depressive' or 'he's a schizophrenic' (patients have an identity outside their illness)
☹ 'you know what so and so (named patient) did'... (guffaws from colleagues in staff canteen). If such behaviour is widespread, it is a toxic workplace and better to find a post where patients are respected and where you feel safe to learn.

****

Figure 18 Sources of Self Help & Aftercare

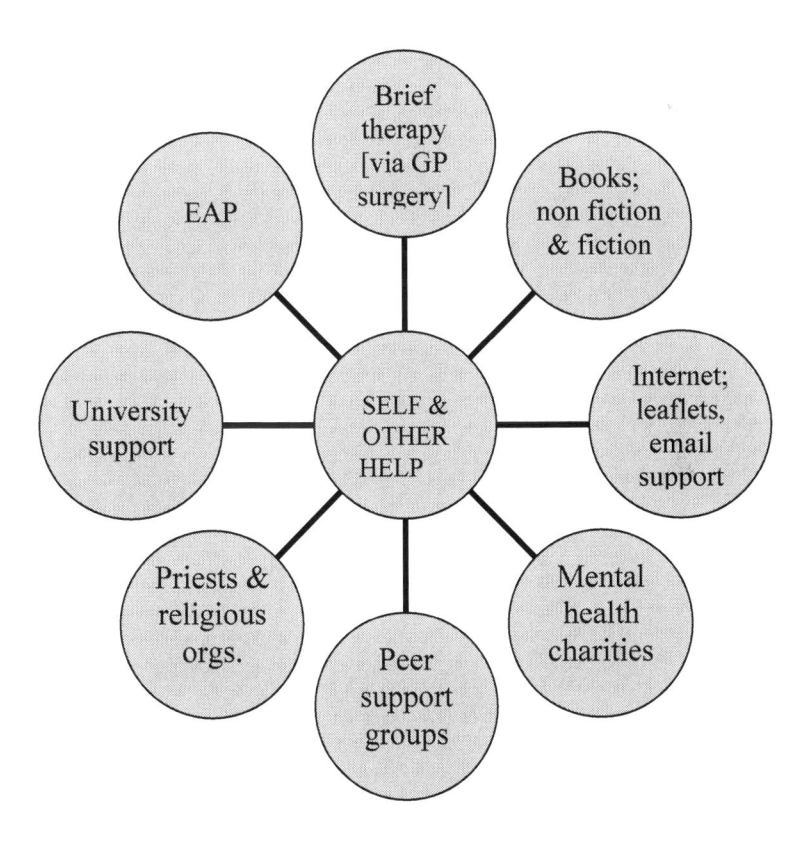

> 'unless you undertake to try to do something beyond what you have already mastered, you will never grow'
> Ronald Osbourne

14   ALTERNATIVE & COMPLEMENTARIES FOR STRESS

Content
Arts therapies
Green & Eco Therapies
Spiritual Therapies – Mindfulness & Meditation
Chinese Herbal Medicine
Healing
Humour Therapy; Gesundheit Institute
Choice of Therapy

There is incredible stress for all those diagnosed with mental illness as well as carers and family. Some of these treatments have been anecdotally found to be effective in relieving stress.

Arts therapies
The Arts therapies are becoming broader ranging and encompass a range of traditional arts:
- art
- music
- drama
- writing and bibliotherapy

The difference between these disciplines expressed as pure art and their use in therapy is interpretation. An art therapist will help the patient interpret what they have drawn; in drama therapy, they will be encouraged to act out archetypal scenes from their life, perhaps with alternative endings being explored. There is as yet no degree in writing therapy but I am sure that will come. Many people have traditionally written diaries, stories, or kept scrapbooks of their lives as a means of reminding themselves of better times or recording their feelings.

Training in art therapies is limited to those who have degrees. There are, I am sure, many people in the community who would make excellent therapists who do not have a Degree, but this is the way the world is going.

Green & Eco Therapies
Green therapies are those which are not based on medical principles, and are connected with the environment. These are growing in popularity as the public lose confidence in drugs for their existential problems. Some enlightened authorities are looking into prescriptions for pets or library

books. There is little evidence base for the effectiveness of such therapies, but plenty of anecdotal or common sense for their use. Reading, pets, walking, climbing and outdoor pursuits, including therapeutic volunteering have long been used for their therapeutic benefit. I covered some of these in more detail in Understanding Mental Illness.

It is clear, as society seeks for respite from stress, for happiness and a new way of life that beneficial exercise or hobbies will become more prominent– if we can somehow find the time to accommodate them. Perhaps one day, like duvet days in the US, we will be allowed time off for relaxation. I am sure this will be beneficial.

Spiritual Therapies – Mindfulness & Meditation

Spiritual therapies and pursuits are more popular in mainstream medicine. Jaded business people and those who work hard bringing up families are seeking that missing something; a gap left by lack of religious life (if we use the model of mind-body-spirit balance). Mindfulness is a simple meditation long used by Buddhists whilst doing daily chores – a simple awareness, concentrating on the task in hand. It sounds simple, but is difficult for those not used to doing one thing at a time. Mindfulness is now very popular in mental health not only for the benefit of patients but also hard-pressed practitioners.

Chinese Herbal Medicine

This is a surprising addition to the NHS, but nevertheless it has been proved effective in a range of situations, from physical to mental illnesses. There are now many Western practitioners as well as those Chinese doctors who have imported their skills and long training to the West. The Chinese have been using natural remedies for centuries. Chinese Herbal Doctors train for years. They use all the parts of a plant – root, bark, stem, leaves, flowers, buds, as well as minerals. The resulting medicines often look strange, smell odd and taste awful but reputedly are effective. The University of Bristol Botanic Garden set up a Chinese herbal garden in 2000 as a joint project with the Register of Chinese Herbal Medicine and this will be used in teaching and research.

Chinese practitioners use a combination of methods including acupuncture, dietary therapy, tai chi or qi gong. Tai Chi is a soft marshal art and qi gong a form of slow but methodical exercise.

Healing

Healing is the most ancient and culturally widespread of therapies – the laying on of hands to affect healing. A popular version is Reiki. There is much anecdotal evidence for the effectiveness of this practice and some scientific evidence. The benefits of a good therapeutic relationship between therapist and patient has long been known, as has the simple matter of human contact. Whilst religious and secular organisations offer courses on healing, there have been natural healers in existence for thousands of years. It will be a shame if this simple folk remedy is over-regulated which will make it hard for people to access.

Humour Therapy; Gesundheit Institute

I could not leave this section without mentioning a controversial therapy which is popular among patients and professional staff. You may have seen the movie Patch Adams; if not, do try to get a copy of it. The movie is the fictionalised version of how Dr Patch Adams set up the Gesundheit Institute. r Adams is a different kind of Doctor who believes in humane health care based on mutuality of interest and shared values. He is also a professional clown, using humour to bring patients to wellness. His team of fellow clown-doctors visit hospitals and clinics world wide to spread their human kindness therapy.

Dr Adams hopes to set up a free hospital; a healing place where professionals and patients live-in on an equal footing. It is a pity he has not yet raised sufficient funds to complete his dream hospital, although he and his supporters have done a great deal of work to that end. Humour is very much on the menu of treatment and as far as possible medication is not used. Mentally ill patients are treated and accepted as they are, even with bizarre symptoms. The few who cannot be treated by the Institute are referred elsewhere. The treatment is not one way but largely an equal healing relationship between professional and patient. Dr Adams hopes patients who come to stay in the hospital will offer other skills to other patients – he cites a mechanic offering to repair cars for those who cannot afford this. This kind of social capital (mutual benefit system) goes beyond medicine into a vision of a new social system. Dr Adams' vision is outside conventional thinking about healthcare but is exactly what his patients ordered. Let me finish with a quotation from Dr Adams:

'Good health [is] deeply related to close friendships, meaningful work, a lived spirituality of any kind, an opportunity for loving service and an engaging relationship to nature, the arts, wonder, curiosity, passion and hope. All of these are time-consuming, impractical needs. When we don't meet these needs, the business of high-tech medicine diagnoses mental illness and treats with pills.'

Comic Relief take note – this is a relevant cause and could do with support outside the US; perhaps a model could be built in the UK?

Choice of Therapy

I was frequently asked about choices by patients who had no prior experience of being in therapy but were tired of medications and pills. They didn't know who to go to for help and found explanations offered by therapists confusing. The best way of helping such dilemmas is by analogy.

This applies whether you are a patient, client or mental health worker advising someone. If you go to a garden centre looking for a plant to fill a gap in your garden, you might find plants you like the look of. So, you read the plant label and see if it will suit the soil, if it likes sun or shade, dry or wet– in other words, if it will **suit the conditions** which you are going to apply to it. It must also suit the plants you already have in place – in other words, it must **fit the environment.** Its no use trying to fit a knot garden in the middle of a cricket pitch. You may also have a budget; if it is tight you are going to hesitate before buying one expensive tree fern – so, it must **suit your pocket**. If you don't like the look, colour or smell of the plant, what is the point of buying it; **go on your instincts** about what is suitable.

Therapy is serious business. It can hurt your pocket more than cure your mind. You might select the wrong therapist a few times but don't stick with them if it's not working.

****

Key Learning
- Arts Therapies – art as therapy involves interpretation of the patient's work, whichever art medium is used.
- Eco & Green Therapies - growing in popularity though rarely funded in the NHS. They include pet therapy, walking, green gym, therapeutic volunteering.
- Spiritual Therapies - have long been used in the East but in Western society are relatively new concepts. Mindfulness meditation is growing in popularity in the NHS.
- Chinese Herbal - based on holistic principles of unity of mind, body and spirit. As well as plant remedies, practitioners use exercise, diet, acupuncture, Tai Chi.
- Humour Therapy; Social Capital - new ways of thinking about healthcare systems, including mutuality and the use of social capital.
- Considering a Therapy - take into consideration; instinct, pocket, evidence, conditions and suitability of purpose.

> 'But it's not magic' said Esk
> 'Most magic isn't.. it's knowing the.. ways of people'
> Terry Pratchett, Equal Rites

15   CASE STUDIES

Content

Emma	Lesley
Alicia	Simon
Joseph	Sandy
Thelma	Soraya

It is difficult for an author to predict how you, as a reader / student of mental health, will want to use a book for learning. There are many ways of presenting materials and it is not always easy to choose which you will enjoy and find useful. I decided to present this material in several ways:
➢ narrative vignettes rather than case studies
➢ diagnoses of major mental illnesses based on DSM IV
➢ explanations for major factors; diagnosis, assessment, confidentiality etc
➢ illustrative diagrams

In my first series Understanding Mental Illness I covered a range of mental illnesses, showing DSMIV and case study equivalents. In a later version I added non-medical treatments with an informal diagnostic exercise. For this book, I decided to tackle it differently. This chapter comprises a series of vignettes to illuminate particular symptoms.

I offer no commentary, diagnostic information nor diagnoses for each vignette. Read the diagnosis section then use this chapter to analyse for yourself what, if anything, is amiss. You will find suggested diagnoses for these vignettes at the end of the chapter on major mental illness.

Remember these vignettes are brief. I have kept out details which a patient might bring to a therapeutic session. I wanted to make it easier, whilst giving a picture of diagnosis and assessment.

It might be useful to **keep a bookmark either end of this block of vignettes** so you can refer back whilst re-reading the chapters on diagnosis and treatment.

****

Note: these are not real people and the vignettes are in no particular order.

Emma

'If I knew I had to go through this again, I would kill myself. I really believed 'they' were following me trying to control my mind. Everyone was in the plot even the doctor and my husband. It was a nightmare - only it was happening during the daytime. I am 40 and was separated after 10 years of marriage. It was not happy. We had no children but looking back I think that was lucky because I would have hated children to go through all this.

My job was awful; a clerical job in a run down office of a housing charity. The Manager hated me and didn't he show it! Tried to get rid of me several times but a nice woman defended me, that is 'til he managed to get rid of her too. There was a drunk manager there too, and he made my life hell.

I can't remember how I ended up in hospital. I think it was Joe, one of my friends. He said I had ignored his calls so he came to my flat. The lights were out but he saw me moving around upstairs. The rest you know. They asked me to describe it, but it was difficult. You know, the whole scenario was so real! I can't remember it coming on, I mean where it changed from me being sane to thinking there were these things in the house from space, trying to take over my mind.

They say that no one remembers this, because it's where you lose insight into the fact that you are getting ill. It was sheer hell. I don't remember how I recovered. I remember bits of reality coming back, as Joe brought bits and pieces to me from home – clothes, books or a few records. I realized that I was 'me' and the things I had thought real did not exist. That was the worst part at first, a real shock – not knowing what was real and what was this awful fantasy. The worst bit was afterwards. I remember the police dragging me into their car and I was screaming. All the bloody neighbours were curtain twitching. That's why I didn't want to go back. Joe sold the place for me and I moved away in the end. I couldn't face the neighbours and the gossip.'

****

Alicia

'I can't remember how it started, but it seemed to be going on for a long time. I was 56 and had been for counselling before but this time I had thought I could cope with Sam's illness. I couldn't respond to friends, but all the time I was saying to myself 'for God's sake don't leave me alone'. Some of them couldn't stand it and deserted me which made it hard, because I started feeling guilty as well, which made it worse.

Mother had had this thing too but I hadn't realized it until I had it myself. She used to spend hours weeping but could never explain why or else she would lie in bed for hours on end, pretending to be asleep if any of us went into her room.

There was no medication or help, so God knows she must have suffered. She tried to kill herself twice and that was awful for us kids. Father didn't know what to do. He left in the end but I suppose I can't blame him.

I don't know what it was with me, genes or my awful marriages. Mother had never been alert enough to be with me so I didn't learn the things a normal teenager would, neither did my sister. We both had several bad marriages and a string of awful boyfriends; nonces and scallywags. Same at work. Always seemed to be picked on.

I don't know what helped in the end. It might have been discovering painting. I know I feel happiest when painting or buying art stuff. I started to exhibit in galleries and gradually found a new life. I married Adrian a few years later. We have a quiet life now. We both like that after all the trauma.'

****

Joseph

'I don't know what mum is worried about. I eat more than any of my friends. Exercise? Yes. I go to the gym every day. If I don't, I feel I've missed out on something. How long? About three or four hours a night. Well, I don't think that's a bit much because some of the real serious guys, the weight lifters, do more than that'.

Joseph is slender with clearly defined muscles; you might say, too clearly defined. What you might notice about him on first sight are his large eyes which slightly dull giving him a sad appearance. Joseph has come to the clinic reluctantly because his parents are worried about him, but he thinks nothing is wrong. It is a hot day but Joseph is wearing a hooded tracksuit top with at least two T-shirts underneath. When the doctor asks him if he wouldn't mind removing the top so that his blood pressure can be taken he reluctantly does so, revealing abnormally thin, though muscular, arms.

'Why do you keep asking about food? I mean, everyone is obsessed about it. What is it with all of you?' Joseph is getting annoyed so the GP changes tack. 'School? Well, school wasn't that good. Some of the teachers were rough. I'd rather not say but we were glad to leave. I don't know what I want. I started in a warehouse because mum needed me to earn something but I hate it. They take everything off you, keep on at you, you know, to do overtime. They dock you for lateness but don't say thanks when you're early or work over.'

'Exams? Well, I did GCSEs. I liked sport and stuff but dad said that won't earn you a crust. Other things? Well, science was ok and maths. I found those easy. I sometimes helped my mates with their homework and they paid me in beer. No, I don't drink a lot. Hey can you leave out this stuff. You promised not to talk about food.'

Joseph is edgy. The Doctor is anxious not to appear threatening because the boy might walk out. This has happened to him before. The Doctor holds up his hands and tells Joseph not to shoot. Joseph laughs and as he does the Doctor notices mottled, yellow teeth with two front ones missing. He makes a note but doesn't say anything.

'No one's asked what I like before. No, not even at school. The teachers didn't like me. They said I was disruptive. I don't know what they meant but I used to get a laugh in class, you know something the teacher said. No, I wasn't happy. I think I was playing clown. Well, sometimes I get a bit down and well, I don't want to talk about it. Is that all? I gotta go.'

The Doctor realizes Joseph is getting edgy so he asks if he will come back for another chat. Joseph says he will, as long as he doesn't mention food. The Doctor says it is a deal and Joseph laughs.

****

Thelma

'It's not me at all, but like a bizarre character from a film. There's no warning, well perhaps a slight feeling of unreality as if everything has got more colour. Every time the pattern is more or less the same. I seem to get into this character that I call her Ameltha because she's a kind of Thelma turned inside out. Ameltha does things that I wouldn't dream of doing.'

Thelma is shy. A librarian-type with round glasses and sensible clothing with flat shoes. Her hair is long and wound into a tight bun. She wears a little makeup but you can tell she is ill. Her eyes are surrounded by dark shadows and her face is too pale. She nervously pulls at threads on her coat. It takes weeks to get the story out. Some weeks she doesn't arrive at the surgery for her appointment and I wonder where she is, what she is doing, who she is being at any given time.

'About six months ago I started drawing money out my savings and putting it in a tin under the bed. It went on for a few weeks. I hadn't been well for a while but no one had noticed because I live alone and my two best friends were away on holiday in Tunisia. I took nearly all of it, nearly £10,000 to a casino in [large hotel]. I dressed up in this red satin suit and high-heels. They were all looking because it left nothing to the imagination. I stayed all night, drinking and chatting up the men. And of course,' she lowered her voice and starts to cry, 'I took a couple up to my room.'

Thelma burst into tears, sobbing for half an hour. I didn't interrupt. She was exhausted. She started again in a very hesitant voice.

'I mean, the money was bad enough but (name withheld) was worse. You see, it wasn't technically rape because I was encouraging them. Or Ameltha was. The things they did.. I was Ameltha and it seemed ok at the time. I thought I was in control, using them. But they were using me. I suppose they look out for women like Ameltha.'

I examine her. She has bruising on her legs and inner thighs. She is torn and I have to stitch her. There are bite marks on her face, neck and shoulders. There are burn marks on her wrists and ankles. I may be a GP but I caught my breath when I saw the scarring on her back and buttocks.

'I can't go to the police. What would I say? As far as I know, there no law that covers it. They would say I consented. Oh yes, I know I could call a Psychiatrist in evidence but what good would that do? I would lose my job.'

She is a professional, respected, a church goer. No one knows about Ameltha not even her two close friends. She laughs and my blood runs cold. That laugh! She is close to the edge.

'Ameltha is ruining me. I can't control her. It.' She starts to scream and then fits. I call the nurse and give her an injection while I call the hospital. The doctor injects her and calls the hospital. She is sectioned.

(A few years later, she is referred again.)

I ask if she has is still taking Lithium. In response, she holds out her hands. They are trembling. Parkinsonism. Lithium is wrecking her nervous system. I ask aloud why else she won't use it because I know that for weeks on end she doesn't.

'It is as if I am nothing without Ameltha. That my life doesn't count. No one notices me. She gives me something, a kind of edge, even though I know the consequences. It's like a drug, this mood. It's as if life suddenly has meaning, that I am the centre rather than being on the tail end. I think that, for a minute or two, I can control the moods but it takes over. I get this feeling of power and confidence but I get frightened and want to back out but it's too late. Ameltha's off to a club. My savings are gone. The house is to be re-possessed. I don't know what to do. My life is not worth living.' Two weeks later, she commits suicide.

****

Lesley

Lesley was cleaning the corners of the window frame with a toothbrush when I arrived. I saw her face from the other side of the window, anxious, red-eyed, almost unaware of her actions. She took a while to answer the door, but when she did, she still had the toothbrush in her hand. Her husband had called the service. He had tried to stop her after several hours but she was still scrubbing away at the imaginary dirt. I could tell he had had enough; he had that look in his eyes. This cleaning had been going on for years and it had worn him down too. I think she realized and that is why she agreed to see me.

It wasn't as if Lesley appeared to have any problems. Nice house, loving husband, two children at University. She had no money worries. Her childhood had been normal and she was higher than average intelligence.

She had told me this a year or more ago. She seemed puzzled at her own behaviour.

'I've tried to stop. Of course I want to. Why do you think I want my fingers to bleed like this? I love Geoff and I know what he is thinking. I don't know what I would do if he left. I know if it doesn't stop that he might.' She picks up a cloth and starts wiping the windowpane, mechanically. 'It's no good asking why. If I knew that, I wouldn't do it. What do I get out of it? Well, the room will be cleaner when I've finished.' We laugh and that breaks the tension.

'I just feel, well, if I don't do it then Geoff and the kids will think I'm being a slob. I don't want that. But it's more than that. I start to feel anxious, stressed really and as soon as I pick up a cloth or duster there's a sort of relief, a calmness.'

The calmness doesn't last more than a minute or two. By then she has started the whole procedure again, top to bottom, the whole house. She can't stop, feels forced to complete her ritual. If she misses a bit, she starts again. Most of the day is taken over with it. She doesn't socialise. Her world is narrowed to this perfectly clean, tidy house she sees as grubby and untidy.

****

Simon

'I wish I knew how it started. It seems ridiculous, especially for a man like me." He chews his fingernail thoughtfully, rapping the fingers of his free hand on his left knee. We are sitting in his cottage, in one of those idyllic villages you see in photographs. He laughed when I said this would be the worst place for him to live in these circumstances. He gestures, encompassing the entire cottage it seems.

'My father's legacy. Nearly half a million. I can't let it go. The property market's depressed.'

I asked if it was that important, money over his mental state. He laughed again but this time it was a cynical laugh. He was moderately wealthy, a playboy and shrewd businessman. He would bring girls here at weekends when his wife was away. I saw him anxiously eyeing beams, cracks in the woodwork.

'At night,' he said. 'It's worse at night. I'm not afraid of anything, but..' His voice tailed off. He was not the sort of man you would want to see on a dark night, I mused. He had an air of something not quite pukka. But he had a problem and I had to cast aside my feelings and try to help.

'So, what is it?' I said after a while.

'It's down to shapes now,' he said. 'Even cracks in the wall. Some of them have fissures. They look like..'

'Spider legs?' I ventured.

He stared at me, eyes narrowing. White-knuckle fear. I could tell he was terrified of losing his reason. It didn't add up for him, how such a small thing can raise terror in a normal, hard headed businessman. To most people it would seem strange, laughable, for a man like him to be afraid of spiders. Some things are not explainable in rational terms but they exist. The mind is a powerful machine and has undercurrents.

****

Sandy

Maude and Arthur are sitting next to me on the threadbare sofa. They are theatricals, film extras with speaking walk-on parts here and there. They make a reasonable living because they are good at what they do. Their daughter Sandy is a worry to them and taints their peace of mind. She was diagnosed when she was 16 and at art school. A talented girl, she was expected to follow family tradition in the creative arts. Now, two years later, she is living a shadowy life in an inner city bedsit, rarely allows visits from her parents or by Social Worker she dislikes (he made the mistake of laughing at her drawings of hallucinatory figures).

'She was always a friendly girl, loved animals, loved her art and drawing. I remember she made a sculpture of her pet dog when she was seven – remember that Arthur?'

Arthur nods, sitting in his armchair sad eyed and quiet. He loves his pretty daughter, was delighted when she got a place at Art College and can't understand what has happened, why she gave up College and is now unemployed and depressed. He can't take in what any of the professionals tell him, particularly when they say there is no cure. He can't get beyond the words 'no cure'.

'We bought her a car to help her be independent but are worried about her driving. We have to keep hoping that she will go back to the Unit if she feels unwell. What if she doesn't take her medication and those things come on?'

'Those things' are hallucinations; frightening visions and voices which terrify Sandy. Once she attacked her father with a chisel cutting his arm so badly he lost the use of several fingers. They refused to press charges even though the policewoman felt it would help; the Courts might give an order so that she received better care.

'She's still my girl,' Arthur suddenly says, with fierce pride, 'she'll find a way through. Made of steel my Sandy.' He still thinks of the other Sandy, the confident girl, not the one living in a twilight, dreamscape world where nightmare and reality are mixed together.

Maude sighs and squeezes Arthur's arm. 'I just don't like the thought of her living up there. I know she can scream and rage and break things when she has delusions but at least we can keep an eye on her. I worry she doesn't eat properly. She likes her grub, my Sandy.' She stifles a sob and Arthur turns to her, kissing her gently on the forehead.

They are getting older, a loving couple who had high hopes for their daughter only to be shattered by this devastating illness. They cannot be sure she is taking vital anti-psychotic medication and are afraid of a relapse. They look at her photograph in a silver frame and start to talk about her younger days. Arthur brightens as he joins in. As they sit there together, under the yellow light from their standard lamps, I can see them as they once were; proper family with a normal family life. I cannot help but feel their loss.

****

Soraya

Soraya is a 30-year old Indian girl. Her family moved to the UK when she was a baby. Apart from the odd holiday they have never returned to the home of their ancestors. However, they still adhere to their culture and beliefs, difficult though it has been for Soraya to accept. Soraya is Westernised and has always attended Western schools. She was brought up to respect her culture but not forced to follow the Muslim faith. She wears Western clothing but keeps her legs covered in the traditional way, more because she is shy and modest than out of tradition. She hoped to find an English boyfriend but her parents forbade it and she daren't disobey. She is afraid of her father and uncles who keep a close watch on her.

For several years since she moved away from home, Soraya has lived alone in a large flat in the suburbs of a city. She has a good job in a bank which earns her a good living. She has plenty of spare cash to spend and could easily go out but chooses to spend much of her time in her flat, where she feels safe and comfortable. Soraya is a worry to her friends from the bank. She has been to some functions and spends her lunch hour with the women, but has never invited any of them to her flat. From what she tells them, Soraya spends a lot of her time reading or watching movies on TV. She is a kind girl but naïve.

Lately, she has been giving a lot of money to charitable causes and wears brighter clothing than usual. She is starting to argue world events with colleagues during lunch hours but before she would sit and eat her food in silence. They have noticed she is eating meat. She was vegetarian but now eats chicken legs, chops and mixed grills from a takeaway around the corner from the bank. Janice, one of her closest colleagues, is concerned. Soraya became angry over something someone said in the canteen and hit the girl with her handbag, burst into tears and rushed out into the street. The men found it funny but Soraya's colleagues were surprised.

Janice, a Supervisor, told the Bank Manager. She felt it was out of character for Soraya. He told her Soraya was starting to make mistakes in her work, which was unusual. They wondered if Soraya had a problem, perhaps a brainstorm. They didn't know what to do and were guessing. Janice suggested they call Soraya in for a chat.

APPENDIX 1 DR SUSAN PARENTI PAPER

Dr Susan Parenti New Model Health Care System For The US
http://www.patchadams.org/re-designing-us-health-care-system/

'The first position is the status quo: the health care system as developed by entrenched health system industries (hospital, insurance, pharmaceutical, information technologies—with government primarily acting as their watchdog). The medical profession of doctor—its history of professional sovereignty—now no longer provides the bottom line in health care. The bottom line belongs to a different bottom: Big Business. We add a third position—whole system design—our frontline, can-do position: **Do it local, do it now, do it small, link with all.**

Given that there's a call for fundamental change in the US health care system, we respond by saying---that means, design something that DOESN'T act like a corporation.

PERTURBATION
Perturbation is the action of desperate and thoughtful people.
Perturbations are ideas/actions that put the system on the spot with the aim of destabilizing it, of making it trip on itself. When thinking of perturbations, we aim at the system's moving itself in a new direction under its own weight and inertia, as it attempts to compensate for our putting it on the spot. This is different from reforming or improving a system, where we aim at ourselves moving the system.

We turn to perturbation when we humbly admit that folks, we're in a David-and-Goliath position here as regards to change of health care system, in that:
1. the system we want to change is in the control of people/institutions who have power over us;
2. the system as is—unchanged—benefits them enormously;
3. these people/institutions have no intention of allowing change of that system, no matter how reasonable and ethical the arguments for change, no matter how compelling the evidence of human suffering and human waste, no matter how many compromises activists are willing to make towards these people/institutions.

In terms of perturbation, we do have a chance: the health care system in the US is so big, so complicated, so bureaucratic, with parts unable to connect to other parts, so insensitive to the mood of its environment, so unable to see its consequences—that falling by means of its own weight is a possibility.

Do we have a choice about anything in health care systems? Yes. Where we have a choice, there we can design.

1. Health care interactions inherit a culture of hierarchy, rank abuse, posing. This is something a group of people, in shaping their health care facility along the lines they want, can support, oppose, change, alter. —this is something that can be designed
2. In our consumerist culture, health/sickness is identified as being an individual property—a person sees her health as her own individual state, she battles against her disease, alone. (This, in the face of many studies that show a person has better health outcomes if she feels her wellbeing integrated within that of a larger group.) A group of healers/designers can come up with a language—frames and metaphors—that oppose this isolationist consumerist tendency, and situate the health of the individual with the health of a group. —this is something that can be designed
3. Health of the staff as important as the health of the patient —this is something that can be designed
4. **Participating in health as a people's popular movement** Commercial culture names a patient as consumer and a doctor/nurse as provider. Given this framing, health care interactions are experienced as a form of shopping, for both patients and healers. Beyond stopping at the counter to get a pill, patients in the United States do not participate in health, health care, or health care systems. Designers can oppose this state of affairs and make elements in their facility (**by means of language, imagery, structure**) that enable popular participation in all aspects/levels of health, health care, and health care system. —this is something that can be designed
5. **Nesting** Currently health care has been nested in bureaucratic and financial institutions. This can be counter-acted: healing interactions need to be protected by nesting them in larger *beneficial* social groups. —this is something that can be designed
6. **Solidarity** We need to rescue the concept/feeling/action of solidarity from North America's garbage heap. In the current culture, each person feels "you're on your own", "everyone for himself". Thus under-staffing of nurses is experienced as the nurses' problem, not the problem of the doctor, medical student, patient, family, technician. This reveals a lack of solidarity between people whose interests are fundamentally in common. This reveals that the lines of solidarity need to be refreshed and redrawn. There need to be discussions about whose interests are being represented. Does the design move in the direction toward creating constructs in which solidarity between the greatest number of different people/groups is supported? —this is something that can be designed
7. **Decision-making** Who makes decisions? Is decision-making about health care system dilemmas communicated to/from the people? Does the

health care system *listen*, in addition to *talk*? —this is something that can be designed

8. **Communication** How is information communicated and disseminated? Where is it? —to be designed

9. **Motivation of actors** Who stands to benefit? In whose interests are decisions made? Are the motivations of the others clear to each? Differences of power? —to be designed

10. Do people seek out health care, or does health care come to them? Is the health care system visible only when a sick person looks for it, or does a person have the sense she is nested in care? —to be designed

11. **Cure or care?** In the health care facility, is there a behaviour which values cure over a commitment to care? —to be designed

12. **Spaces** Does the space (rooms, hallways, waiting rooms) support the values we want? —to be designed

13. **Presentation of self in everyday life** The way healers, staff, and patients act in everyday life is a choice and can be a tremendously valuable input to desirable health care interactions. There is no neutral interaction. —to be designed

The health care crisis is, amongst other things, a crisis of bankrupt ideas. People recognize that things need to change; they do not recognize that something has to be *made up*.

THE ANSWERS

Systems are circular; something which seems to be a cause turns out to be an effect of something else, and so on. Where to start?

If a system of **one payer, single tier, universal access** is created, then hopefully that will lead to a significant change in many other aspects of the culture of care in the system.

Designs where the **health care relation *shapes* the system, and where the system *protects* the relation**. If a group of health care providers at a clinic are involved in designing their practice, our hope is that a change in the culture of care will open the way to a change in the funding of it, or at least make people more susceptible to that change.

We say—local initiatives for the good of the public renew the sense of confidence in a group of people governing. **Campaign universally, design locally.**

Our strategy is this—rather than priding ourselves in working with organized business, we want to oppose and **expose the undesirability of market-controlled health care** and to **popularize a hands-off-health care**, corporations!! sentiment in Americans and in business-people themselves.

The abundance of bureaucracy in the medical system—the paperwork, the overseeing of diagnostic decisions by insurance companies, etc.—is not an error in the system. It is the *intended consequence* of the current system. **The system is being maintained at the expense of the well being of its members**.

Talking Points
1. We question at every opportunity the appropriateness of market capitalism to control (nest) the delivery of health care. We discuss the limits of free markets and the need for non-market regulation of experiential goods (a term in economics for services whose outcome is uncertain). We point out that in the case of a relationship dominated good such as health care, cutting costs in overhead results in cutting care itself.
2. We debate the assumption that health care is (needs must be) expensive. The expense of health care is not a property of health care in itself; the expense is an engineered condition, a consequence of the present design. We debunk the framing that health care will always be costly by making reference to counter-examples.
We invite media and wireless activists to demonstrate how the use of technology in health care can be free.

Every time the question, "Who will pay for this expensive system" is asked, we balance this with our question, "Who has been profiting such that this system is expensive?"

Health care, by its nature, is inexpensive—it's primarily a relationship along with some tools. We keep that image in mind so that we avoid playing into the assumptions of the market. The "high cost of care", the "complexity of the system" are frames that fuel the symbolic capital of the current system.
3. We caution that when big business says "we're committed to cutting costs in health care" this DOES NOT mean "we're committed to making health care inexpensive". It doesn't mean that. Within market capitalism cutting costs means lowering overhead (workers' wages, resources) to keep profit at margins attractive to investment capital. It *does not* refer to lowering the cost of health care so that it's easily available to us who need it. Market forces always say they want to cut costs; the question of reducing their profit margins is never brought up.
4. We rename the health care system the 'disease management system'. When a person gets into the medical system, that person is getting disease management not health care. Disease management is a far smaller domain than the domain of health care. Health care is a huge domain of interactions, happening primarily outside the medical system, available to all, only not organized. John Glick, MD says, "Every moment is a health care moment". When does health care start? — when you decide to take a walk early in the morning? When you feel like you're getting a cold and a friend gives you Echinacea drops in a cup of tea?

What is health care at its indispensible minimum? Against the noise tunnel of the expensive and complicated disease management system we need to keep in mind the simplicity of a desirable health care relation: it's a bi-directional relation of care, always available, always findable—as a matter of fact you don't have to look for it, it looks for you. One has a sense of being inside caring, of being nested in care—there's someone to turn to, to talk to, they suggest a few things to do, you do them, you turn to them again.

The protection of this simple relation, of its friendly permeating steadfast thoughtful presence, is the primary function of any system/culture built around it. Thus the system/culture would be so designed that this relation is either freely offered or offered at a low cost (supported by communal and social structures in a variety of ways); that the formation of any bureaucracy around it would be a sign of malfunctioning or predators, and steps would be taken to eliminate that; that creativity and variety would go into the design of the supporting nest into which the relation is put, and into the relation itself. So einfach.

5. Do we attempt to work with market institutions to change health care? Organized business is interested in discussing financing and administration, not health or health care. Thus, to sit down at the table with these major players in health care industries means to sit down with people who frame every discussion of health/health care as a discussion of money and administration. If any other consideration is brought up, they will look at you with a patronizing eye—after all, they know their business—and turn it back into a discussion of financing. So we *can* sit down with them at the table, but we have to realize we're sitting down with opponents to any direction of creating a desirable health care system available to all.

6. We need to garner support from business people, on a person-by-person basis, for hands-off-health-care initiatives. To appeal to faith communities whose morals lead them to ethical political positions. Every businessman has his fatherhood looking over his shoulder; has his son-hood, brotherhood. Every businesswoman is also a mother, daughter, sister, friend. Do they want to overhear, in the waiting room, that cutting costs was a factor in why their grandchild died on the operating table? At some point in their lives, someone they care about will be in the system too. Their own pricey insurance policies cannot be transferred to everyone they care about.

7. We consider what is happening to health care in the US a local version of the same market theories that initiated Structural Adjustment Programs across the globe by WTO and World Bank. (Structural adjustments' primary focus is to shape institutions/countries so that they're attractive to long distance investment capital.)

Structural adjustment policies have been tried in South America, and met, in an increasing number of cases, with resistance. Let's link our resistance to structural adjustment policies at home to the resistance made by allies across the globe who are also fighting these policies.

Final Remarks

The components of what we're calling 'Whole System Design' are two calls: one is a call for a variety of designs of those elements that will be become the culture of health care; and the second is a call for the sentiment: "hands off health care, big business" to become infectious in the Americas. Both these calls are efforts to perturb the current system.

In 2006, people in the United States have a diagnosis of the problem of our health care system that is clear and intelligent. If you read blogs/letters/emails from the common person they articulate their discontent with the health care system in a sophisticated way. (See membership polls conducted in spring, 2006, by MoveOn.Org). People want a fundamental change in the health care system. This means, we want a change in the fundamentals.

We need to be prepared for the language/framing in response to this desire for change. When Medicare Plan D came out in May 2006, it was a 122-page document with lots of complicated sections, written for older Americans, telling them how to get pharmaceutical drugs. 122 pages? Huh? How was this allowed? Did the writers lack schooling, lack funding, lack time to do a better job? We don't think so. Plan D was a linguistic display of 'passive intervention'.

We need to watch out. The existing players (entrenched industries, along with their current protectorate: the government) will respond to our clear desire for fundamental change with an engineered Tower of Babel. The column of language is coming at us now: fundamental change in the health care system is re-framed as the question "who will pay for this expensive system?" as a debate between various complicated payment schemes, as a mandate for consumer choice. 'Universal insurance' will be used, to confuse us into thinking this means 'single payer'. The language will befuddle us, discourage us.

The temptation will be to leave the discourse around health care to the experts. They seem to know what they're talking about, right? None of these experts will challenge the structural power of the entrenched industries, the huge salaries of the health care corporations CEO's, the fact that pharmaceutical corporations top the chart for profit returns, etc.

Will we permit 'passive intervention', again? The statistic is cited, over and over again, that in the richest country in the world, nearly 48 million Americans do not get health care.

We say that in the richest country in the world, 300 million Americans do not get health care. Yes, of these 300 million, many people do get into the disease management bureaucracy, as they have insurance. But what is happening inside the medical system is no longer care; the 567,000 licensed doctors are not permitted to doctor; the 2.4 million nurses are being thwarted at nursing. The culture of health care in America is being morphed into something else.

When hospitals and clinics are businesses, and doctors/nurses become business people, who will we then turn to for health care?

November, 2006" [Dr Susan Parenti]

****

GLOSSARY
A

actualization	self-improvement
acupuncture	Chinese treatment - re-balancing energy
adenine	one of four 'building blocks' of DNA
agoraphobia	fear of open spaces
alternative medicine	alternative to conventional medicine
altruistic	generosity of spirit
Analytical Psychology	psychological therapy [Carl Jung]
ancestor worship	culture of venerating dead ancestors
anhedonia	inability to experience happiness
anorexia nervosa	eating disorder; restricting food intake
antidepressant	drug reducing symptoms of depression
antimanic	drug reducing symptoms of mania
antipsychotic	drug - reduces psychosis
anxiety	Unpleasant emotional arousal
arachnophobia	fear of spiders
archetype	character trait in personality (Jung)
armouring	physical tensions in body [Reich]
arts therapy	therapy using art, music or drama
Assertive Outreach	teams working to prevent patient relapse
assessment	diagnosis by non medical therapists
Asylum	Victorian institute for insane
auto hypnosis	self hypnosis; a deep relaxation
avoidance	deliberately avoiding fearful situation

B

BAC	British Association for Counselling
balanced personality	balance of mind, body, spirit
Bedlam [historic term]	Uproar; originates from Bethlem
behaviour	way we react to situations
behaviour pattern	consistent reaction
behavioural therapy	therapy aimed at modifying behaviour
Bethlem or Bedlam	second oldest Hospital in England
bi-polar	illness; alternating depression and mania
bile (black bile)	one of 4 supposed elements humours
binge eating or binging	uncontrolled eating and purging
blood/infection phobia	fear of blood, or infection by needles
BPS	British Psychological Society
brain chemistry	chemicals produced by transmitters
brain fever	(historic) psychosis
brain scan	electrical activity in the brain
Breuer Joseph	Victorian hypnotist

brief psychotic disorder	mental illness brought on by stress
Brief therapy	time limited therapies
British Association for Counselling [BAC]	umbrella organisation for counselling and psychotherapy
Buddhism	teaching of Gautama Buddha
bulimia	eating disorder, purging and vomiting

C

care plan	document, outlining care for patient
case history	psychological and physical history
case notes	records kept by therapists
Computerised Axial Tomography [CAT]	computer scan of whole body; uses scan put together by computer
catatonia	mental state - lack of movement
Catharsis or cathexis	Greek for purging; 'letting go'
Charcot Jean Martin	famous Victorian hypnotist
'checking and testing'	compulsive; excessive checking
chemical imbalance	chemicals; serotonin or dopamine
chemical transmitter	way brain chemicals are distributed
Chemist	scientist trained in medications
Chinese herbal medicine	herbs, Tai Chi, acupuncture, exercise
Citizenship [curriculum]	New addition to national curriculum
claustrophobia	fear of confined spaces
client-centred therapy	Rogerian unconditional positive regard
Clinical guidelines	standards or rules fie clinical work
Clinical Psychologist	psychologist in medical setting
clinical responsibility	legal responsibility for patient
clinical trial	testing of new drugs
clinician	person who practices medicine
CMHT	Community Mental Health Team
cognition	to recognise
cognitive-behavioural therapy [CBT]	therapy for recognition and change of poor behaviour patterns
Collective unconscious	ancestor or cultural myths [Jung]
complementary therapies	therapies not based on medical theory
compliance (of patient)	extent to which patients willingly take prescribed drugs
compulsion	urge to carry out a certain act or ritual
computer modelling	models of body using computers
conditioned response	behaviour depends upon stimulus
conflict (mental)	two or more opposing events/ beliefs
conscious (mind)	part of the mind aware of its actions
contra-indication	one substance which affects another

copyright	law forbidding plagiarism
Coroner	Officer investigates unnatural deaths
Francis Crick	one of 4 DNA pioneers see also Franklin R, Watson J, Wilkins M
crippled	(historic) physically disabled
Crown Prosecution	body which decides on criminal cases
crystal healing	healing by placing crystals on body
cytosine	one of protein 'building blocks' DNA

D

de ja vue	memory of reliving a past event
de-sensitising	therapeutic exposure to fear
delusion	ideas perceived as real
dementia	irreversible brain damage
demon	devil or evil spirit
depot injection	monthly injection, in buttocks or thigh
'depressive'	(derogatory) depressive illness
depressive illness	Mental Illness of intense hopelessness
diagnosis	deducing illness from observation
Diagnostic & Statistics V	manual for diagnosing mental illness
Divine retribution	punishment by gods for mortals
DNA	genes
drug trial	Research of drug's effectiveness
drugs	medications; colloquial for illegal drugs
DSM (V)	see ' Diagnostic & Statistics Manual'

E

eating disorder	illness -restricting food intake
eco therapy	green therapy – green gym, walking etc
Electro Convulsive Therapy (ECT)	electric shock treatment given to treat depression or schizophrenia
electric eels	(historic) treatment for madness
electro-encephalograph [EEG]	reading on a printed tape or monitor of electrical brain activity
empathy	understanding of personal feelings
epigram	short quotation
epilepsy	interruption of electric flow to brain
episodic [mental illness]	periods of mental illness
Erickson, Milton	pioneer of brief therapies
ethical	moral code
euphoria	extremely intense high mood
evidence-based medicine	medicine proven through research
evil spirits	imagined entity blamed for madness

existential	the area of human existence
extrovert	outgoing, confident personality

F

forensic psychiatry	criminal mental illness psychopathic
fragmenting	experience of psychosis
Rosalind Franklin	one of 4 DNA pioneers see also Crick F, Watson J, Wilkins M.
Frankl Viktor	Famous Jewish Psychiatrist
free association	method for unlocking unconscious
Freud Sigmund	founder of psycho analysis

G

Galen	ancient Greek Doctor
Gestalt	unifying therapy
Green therapy	see eco
Group Home	homes for ex- patients living together
group therapy	Therapy with many patients
Guanine	one of four proteins of DNA

H

Hallucination, auditory	unreal voices or sounds
hallucination - visual	seeing things which are not real
Haloperidol	medication to treat mania
healing	simple folk remedy
herbal medicine	Chinese therapy using plants
hero	Jungian archetype - hero myth
'high'	exaggerated emotion
Hippocrates	Greek Philosopher and Doctor
holistic therapy	Tri part Eastern belief
homeopathy	diluted herbs which mimic symptoms
Humanistic therapy	therapy based on ethical thinking
humour or 'vital fluid'	ancient medicine, 4 life-giving fluids
Hypno-Psychotherapy	brief therapy using hypnosis
hypnosis	bypassing conscious by relaxation
hypnotic state	state of relaxation [see trance]
hypothesis	initial assumption made in research;
hysteria	(historic)- high emotional state
hysterical paralysis	(historic) paralysis from mental state

I

Idiot [historic]	incapable of making decisions.
Imax	huge screen which shows 3D movies

impulse	powerful desire to do or act out
individuation	Jungian – integration of personality
Inquisition	17th century church-based court
insanity (historic)	mental processes not functioning
insight	ability to understand situation
institutionalisation	deterioration of independence
introvert	thinking, inward looking personality
isolation	separated from community

J

Jung Carl	founder of Analytical Psychology
Jungian Analyst	follower of the Jungian school

L

Laing R. D.	'myth of mental illness' Psychiatrist
Largactil	Early form of anti psychotic medicine
lay person	someone not formally
Lazar or leper house	Institutional home for lepers
leucotomy (lobotomy)	psychosurgery, cutting frontal lobes
libido	sexual energy
librium	tranquilliser see also 'valium'
'life event'	Vivid event remembered
lithium	natural but dangerous metallic salt
lobotomy	see leucotomy
lunatic (historic)	insane; belief moon caused madness

M

mad (historic)	old term for mental illness
Mania or manic	mental illness of frantic moods
maniac	(historic) – mad person
massage	manipulation of muscles by pressure
medical model	theory of medicine i.e. medications
medication	drugs to cure or alleviate symptoms
meditation	peaceful contemplation
melancholia	(historic) depressive illness
Mental Health Act 1983	Defunct law for sectioning insane
Mental Health Tribunal	empowered to detain/ release patients
Mental Health Worker	similar to Rehabilitation Officer
mental illness	illness of the mind
Mental Nurse	Worker qualified to administer drugs
Milton Erickson	US Psychiatrist, father of brief therapy
MIMS	manual of drugs and characteristics
Mind	national mental health charity

mindfulness	Buddhist meditation of awareness
model	pattern or opinion or simulation
modelling (of humans)	Diagrams, theories to explain
mood swings (rapid)	rapid mood change e.g. mania
moral panic	short lived community concern
music therapy	art therapy using music

N

Natl. Health Service	Nye Bevan's public healthcare
Natl. Inst. of Clinical Excellence [NICE]	provides evidence based research for medical treatments
nervous breakdown	slang for brief psychotic disorder
neuro transmitters (brain)	nerve cells with chemical messengers
NLP	neuro-linguistic programming; brief therapy
noradrenaline	chemical (see also serotonin)
normal	'that which most people accept'
normalizing	making a condition acceptable

O

obsession	preoccupation
obsessive-compulsive disorder [OCD]	mental illness of obsessions and compulsions, leading to rituals
Osteopathy	therapeutic manipulation of spine

P

P [medication packs]	pharmacist present when dispensed
paedophile	male sexually attracted to children
panic attack	fear, onsets without warning
paranoia	extreme psychological fear
paranoid schizophrenia	form of schizophrenia
Parkinson's Disease [Parkinsonism]	disease characterised by tremors or drug induced muscular tremor
Patch Adams, Dr	US Psychiatrist of humour therapy
Pathology [pathological]	showing signs of illness
Pavlov, Ivan Petrovich	Neurologist of conditioned response
perception	A way of understanding
Personality	The personal qualities of self
pharmaceutical	relating to drugs industry
pharmaceutical drugs	synthetic materials or plants as drugs
Pharmacist	scientist who works with drugs
phobia	deep-rooted fear e.g. spider, flying, dirt
placebo	inert medication part of drug trial tests
Plato	Greek Philosopher who studied mind

POM	prescription only drugs
Project Atlas (WHO)	mapping health resources world-wide
Prozac	SSRI drug for depression
psyche	Greek goddess representing the soul
Psychiatrist	Doctor qualified in psychiatric drugs
psychiatry	treatment / study of mental disorders
psycho	(modern derogatory) insane.
psycho analysis	therapy by Sigmund Freud
Psycho Analyst	therapist; practices psycho-analysis
psycho-dynamic	understanding personal relationships
psycho-educational	training e.g. stress management
psychodrama	therapy 'acting out' patient's life
psychological makeup	essence of personality
psychology	study of human behaviour
psychopath	personality disorder; absent conscience
psychosis	out of touch with reality
psychosurgery	brain surgery
psychosynthesis	therapy integrating the self
Psychotherapist	Therapist; enabling insights

R

reductive	something explained without full facts
reflect	to consider something deeply
Rehabilitation Officer	therapist of mental health patients
Rehabilitation Units	modern social care unit
Reich, Wilhelm	founder of Reichian Therapy
Reiki	method of healing by touch
Rogers, Carl	founder of client-centred therapy
Royal College of Psychiatrists	UK professional body of Psychiatrists

S

St John's Wort	herb, useful in treatment of depression
sanity	distinguish between real & imagined
scapegoat	sacrificed animal or person
schizophrenia	illness with delusions, hallucinations
School of Thought	method of training
Social Care Institute for Excellence [SCIE]	provides evidence based research on social care [values based]
'section' / 'sectioning'	slang - detained - Mental Health Act
self hypnosis	voluntary state of deep relaxation
serendipity	accidental discovery
serotonin	chemical transmitter

Shaman	priest, North American Indian culture
shiatsu	Japanese massage using fingertips
ship of fools	16th century cure for lunacy
Harold Shipman [MD]	GP serial killer. Murdered 15 patients
Skinner, Burrus Frederic	scientist - behavioural theory
side effect	unwanted effects of drugs
Situational phobia	fear of situations e.g. lifts, aeroplanes
Social Care Institute for Excellence [SCIE]	evidence based research for social care
social phobia	fear of social situations
solution-focused therapy	brief therapy; solutions to problems
Spanish Inquisition	medieval -delegated to try witches
'speaking in tongues'	'babbling'- 'voices of God'
SSRI's	specific Serotonin Re-Uptake Inhibitor; antidepressants
Standard[s]	Written basis of care or treatment
stigma or stigmatise	negative opinion fuelled fear
Stimuli	perceive by senses
stress	forces which determine action
sub personality	individual characteristic (see archetype)
subconscious	Ancient part of mind
Suicide Act 1961	act making it illegal to assist suicide
supervision	learning through discussing patients with experienced therapist
symbolic insight	as in dreams; learning from symbols
synthesised/ synthesis	combining chemicals as new drugs
Thomas Szaz	Psychiatrist of social construct

T

Tai Chi	Chinese exercise and soft martial art
Temple of Light	ancient Roman cure for melancholia
Therapeutic Community	community of patients and therapists
Thinking pattern	habitual way of thinking
Thorndike, Edward	Behaviourist - reward & punishment
Thought disorder	problems with linear thinking
thymine	one of four proteins of DNA
trance	deep relaxation bypassing unconscious
tranquilliser or 'tranny'	drug which suppresses nervous system
trepanning	primitive psycho-surgery

U

unconditional positive	Rogerian therapy

regard	
unconscious	hidden from awareness
uncovered	therapy term - discovery

V

valium	addictive tranquilliser
virtual drug trial	testing drugs using computers
virtual brain	computer model of human brain
visualisation	imagining event to help it become real
vital fluids	see 'humour'
voodoo	cult practised in Haiti connected with the raising of the dead for rites

W

Watson, James	one of 4 DNA pioneers see also Crick F, Francis R, Wilkins M
Watson, John Broadus	Psychologist of behavioural theory
White Paper	proposals for new legislation
Wilkins, Maurice	one of 4 DNA pioneers see also Crick F, Francis R, Watson J
Witch	ancient term; human servant of devil
Witchcraft	practice of magic for good or evil
'word salad'	meaningless strings of words manifested in schizophrenia
World Health Organisation (WHO)	consortium of many countries who come together to improve standards in health care

FURTHER READING

The following are in alphabetical order by subject.

THE ARTS ON LIFE

Paintings by   **William Blake**
An artist who successfully portrays madness and suffering

The Plains of Heaven   **John Martin**
One of a trilogy about The Day of Judgement

One Flew Over the Cuckoos Nest   movie
Now made into an award-winning movie, the book is a fictional account about lobotomy. Although overstated it does give some idea of the tragedy of Asylums.

Shine   movie
Based on the true story of concert pianist David Helfgott who had a nervous breakdown but later married and came back to the concert hall

A Beautiful Mind   movie
Based on the true story of mathematician Dr John Nash, diagnosed with schizophrenia, he later became a Nobel prize winner

Rain Man   movie
Based on the true story of autistic savant Kim Peek

BIOGRAPHIES/DIARIES - mental illness

Kay Redfield Jamison   **An Unquiet Mind**
Dr Jamison's own experience of manic-depressive illness

Jacki Lyden   **Daughter of the Queen of Sheba**
Jacki's mother was diagnosed with mania and almost destroyed the lives of her family

RESEARCH & HISTORY OF MENTAL ILLNESS

Roy Porter   **A Brief History of Madness**
An easy-to-read history of mental illness and its treatment.

American Psychiatric   **DSM IV**
Association
The diagnostic manual used by psychiatrists world wide to diagnose mental illness. See also websites

J Andrews, J Briggs et al   **The History of Bethlem**

A history of the earliest of the Asylums.

Sainsbury Centre for Mental   **Beyond the Water Towers**
Health
Up to date expert papers on aspects of the treatment of mental illness, from asylums to the present day. Very readable.

CASE STUDIES & THERAPIES

Malcolm Macmillan   **An Odd Kind of Fame:**
                                         Stories of Phineas Gage

The author is a well-known psychiatrist, This book is about the Victorian man who's accident inspired research into the functional areas of the brain, and also the infamous lobotomy.

Oliver Sacks   **The Man Who Thought His**
                                         Wife Was a Hat
The author is a well-known psychiatrist who writes interesting vignettes about aphasia, an illness which prevents patients properly translating what they see.

Virginia Axline   **Dibs, in Search of Self**
How a lost child was brought back into the world by a Psychotherapist.

Dr Kay Redfield Jamison   **Touched with Fire**
A book covering the them of manic depression and creativity.

Carl Rogers   **Client-Centred Therapy**

Carl Rogers famous book about his humanistic therapy.

INTERESTING WEBSITES

Complementary Medicine
http://www.baat.org/
British Art Therapy Association

http://www.acupuncture.org.uk
British Acupuncture Council

http://www.bcp.org.uk/
British Psychoanalytic Council

http://www.bamt.org/
British Society for Music Therapy

http://www.bwy.org.uk/
British Wheel of Yoga

http://www.mctimoney-college.ac.uk/
McTimoney Chiropractic

http://www.homeopathy-soh.org/
Society of Homeopaths

http://www.rchm.co.uk/
The Register of Chinese Herbal Medicine

Medication

http://www.rcpsych.ac.uk/healthadvice/treatmentswellbeing/antidepressants.aspx
Royal College of Psychiatrists factsheet on antidepressants

http://www.hospitalclown.com/
A kind of medication for those who dare to be different.

Mental Health Organisations

http://www.depressionalliance.org/
Mental health generally

http://www.samaritans.org.uk/know/statistics.shtm
Samaritans on-line

http://www.sane.org.uk/
SANE & saneline (helpline) mental health charity website

http://www.rethink.org/
Rethink (formerly National Schizophrenia Fellowship) mental health charity

http://www.depressionalliance.org/
The Depression Alliance mental health charity

http://www.retreat-hospital.org/
The Retreat hospital. Care for anyone with mental health problems (York Retreat)

www.turning-point.co.uk
Turning Point, for mental health rehabilitation & counselling

www.mind.org.uk
MIND, the mental health charity

http://www.depressionalliance.org/
Depression alliance mental health charity

Science & Technology

https://www.imax.com/countries/gb/
Imax cinema

New Discoveries about Psychosis
http://www.bbc.co.uk/news/uk-wales-south-east-wales-34508014

Training
http://www.rgu.ac.uk/subj/pharmacy/pharmacy.htm
School of Pharmacy web site

http://www.hull.ac.uk/home/prospectus/undergrad/social_work.html
Training in Social Work

http://www.uncommon-knowledge.co.uk/milton_erickson/family_therapy.html
http://www.creativity.co.uk/creativity/guhen/erickson.htm
About the founder of all brief therapies - Dr Milton Erickson

http://www.newtherapist.com/20hitch.html
an amusing journey through brief therapy, in metaphorical style

OTHER

"One child, one teacher, one book, one pen can change the world."
Malala Yousafzai, Education Campaigner
http://www.bbc.co.uk/news/magazine-24379018

Story of Patty Hearst.
http://www.biography.com/people/patty-hearst-9332960

INDEX

A Beautiful Mind - movie 149
Action for Relatives 38
Aftercare 103
Analytical Psychologist 77
Analytical Psychology .... *See* also C G Jung
Anorexia 50
Arts therapies 119
Assertive Outreach 104
Asylum Patients 7, 105
Behavioural Therapy 81
Brief Psychotic Disorder 47
BRIEF PSYCHOTIC DISORDER 47
C G Jung 19, 81
cannibal 13
Case History 35, 39, 44
CASE STUDIES 123
Causes of Mental Illness 20
CBT diagram 83
Change In Behaviour 37
Changes in Appearance, Hygiene or Weight 37
Changes In Mood 37
Chinese Herbal Medicine 120
Choice of Therapy 121
Clinical Nurse Specialist 102
Clinical Psychologist 78
Cognitive Behavioural Therapy 82
Columbine High School 13
Commonality of Experience 28
Commonality of Mental Illness 19, 26
Community attitudes 22
Compulsion 53
Confidentiality 67, 69, 72
Continuum - Mental Health to Illness 29
Counselling Charitable Organisations 106
Counsellor 78
Country of the Blind 13
Criminality & Mental Illness 13, 14
Crown Prosecution Service 35
Cultural Factors 43, 45
Cultural issues 22
Danger of Making Assumptions 41

Decision-making	132
Define Insanity	17
Degrees	68
depot injection	72, 141
DEPRESSIVE ILLNESS	48
Diagnosis	1, 5, 26, 35, 40, 41, 43, 44, 45, 46
Diagnosis - aim of	43
Diagnosis - stages	44
Diagnostic Exercise - answers	60
Diagnostic Manual DSMV	45
Disagreements over training changes yr 2000	93
DNA	21, 35, 139, 141, 142, 146, 147
do sanity and insanity exist	16
Does Insanity exist	16
Dr Aubrey de Grey	23
Dr Harold Shipman	13, 23, 74, 146
Dr John Nash	48, 57
Dr Milton Erickson	76, 81, 89, 143, 153
Dr Patch Adams	121
DR SUSAN PARENTI	131
DSMV	45, 46
Early signs of mental illness	35, 38
EATING DISORDERS	49
Encounter Groups	87
Evidence-Based Care	73, 79
Experiencing the Dead	58
Family Work	90
Finding Identity in Large Organisations	95
Force-feeding	50
Fragmentation of Personality	58
Free to Roam	35
General Practitioners	70
George Berkeley	16
Gestalt	87
Graduate Mental Health Worker	93, 102
Green & Eco Therapies	119
Group Behaviour in Change Situations	97
Hallucinations	47
Haloperidol	17, 112, 142
Healing	120
Hospitalising Without Sectioning	39
Humour Therapy; Gesundheit Institute	121
Hypno-Psychotherapist	75

Hypno-Psychotherapy 88
Imax Cinema 57
Informal Rules For Mental Health Workers 115
Knowledge and Skills Framework 100
Leadership Models 94
Lewin's Unified Field Theory 99
Lithium 44, 143
Making changes - diagram 95
Malala Yousafzai 22
MANIA 50
Masters Degree 96
Medical Practitioner 67, 68
Medication in Mental Health 112
Mental & Physical Examination 44
Mental Illness Difficult to Spot 36
MIMS 45
Mindfulness & Meditation 120
Modelling 85
moral codes 13
Moral Panics 7, 15
Movies about mental illness 149
National Institute for Health & Clinical Excellence (NICE) 111
National Occupational Standards (NOS) 101
NHS Reform 93, 94
Obsession 53
OBSESSIVE COMPULSIVE DISORDER (OCD) 52
Occupational Therapist (OT 74
OCD 31, 47, 52, 53, 62, 144
One Flew Over the Cuckoos Nest 149
Over Reacting 37
Parallel Experience 31
Perceptions 22
PERTURBATION 131
Pharmacists 71
phobia 43, 54, 81, 139, 144, 146
PHOBIA 54
Placebo 109, 112
Prochaska and DiClemente's trans-theoretical model 95
Psychiatrists 70
Psycho Analyst 76
Psychology 67, 78, 81, 84, 86, 90, 91, 95, 139, 143
psychopathic personality disorder 13, 16, 59
Psychopathic Personality Disorder 59

psychosis... 17, 18, 22, 31, 45, 47, 48, 50, 56, 57, 104, 112, 114, 139, 142, 145
Psychotherapist 77
Qualities of Therapists 73
Quality Control in Therapies 110
Rain Man - movie..149
Reasons for Non-Arrival of Patients 40
Registered Mental Nurses..72
Rehabilitation Units 104
Rehabilitation Worker (Rehab.) 74
Reichian Therapy 90
Rogerian therapy 88
SCHIZOPHRENIA..56
Schizophrenia - Catatonic..59
Schizophrenia - Paranoid...59
Schools of Thought 81, 85
Self Help 106
Self Help - sources 117
Shine - movie 149
Sigmund Freud 76
Social Care Centre for Excellence (SCIE) 111
Social Worker...75
Solitude 61
Solution-Based (Brief) Therapy 89
Stockholm Syndrome 17
Stress 5, 22, 24, 26
Support for Day Patients 104
Support for Enduring Mental Illness...104
Systematic De-sensitisation ....*See* also Behavioural Therapy
Talking Cures...84
Therapeutic Communities 7, 103, 106, 107, 108
Therapeutic Relationship 112
Thought Disorder and 'Word salad' 58
Trades v Professions 98
Tribunal 36, 143
Tuckman Model - group behaviour 97
Types of Treatment - diagram 63
Who Are the Best Therapists..74
Why Do We Become Analytical 28
Wilhelm Reich 90
Withdrawal or Marked Change to Usual Routine......................................37

Figure 19 Social Problems of Mental Illness

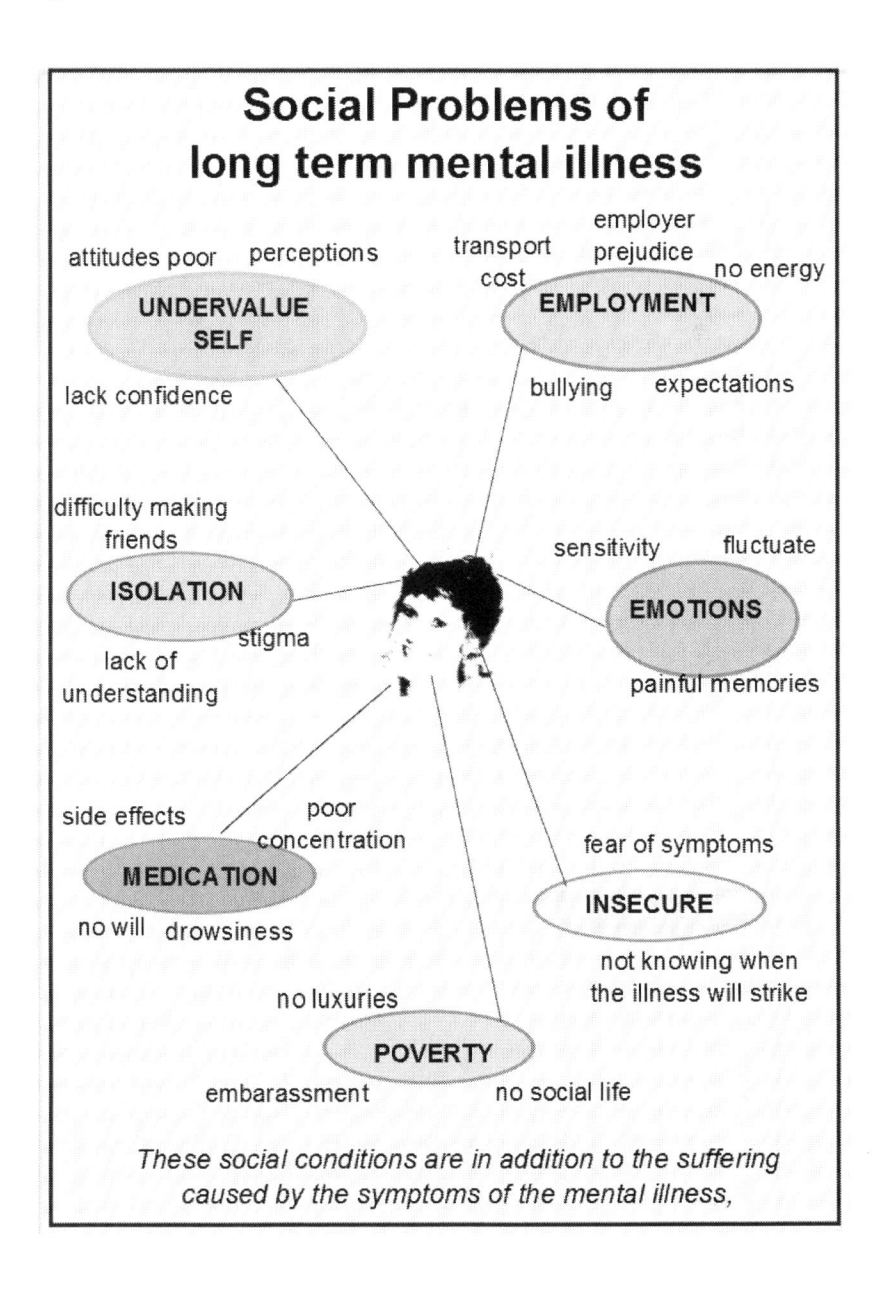

Social Problems of long term mental illness

UNDERVALUE SELF
- attitudes poor
- perceptions
- lack confidence

EMPLOYMENT
- transport cost
- employer prejudice
- no energy
- bullying
- expectations

ISOLATION
- difficulty making friends
- stigma
- lack of understanding

EMOTIONS
- sensitivity
- fluctuate
- painful memories

MEDICATION
- side effects
- poor concentration
- no will
- drowsiness

INSECURE
- fear of symptoms
- not knowing when the illness will strike

POVERTY
- no luxuries
- embarassment
- no social life

These social conditions are in addition to the suffering caused by the symptoms of the mental illness.

Printed in Great Britain
by Amazon